The Complete Family Guide

Navigating the Journe

Surviving Schizophrenia Workbook and Manual for Families and Individuals

Joann Rose Gregory

"Embrace the journey, even when it's hard. Remember, in the heart of every challenge lies an opportunity for growth. With patience, understanding, and unwavering hope, we can navigate the waves of schizophrenia together."

Joann Rose Gregory

Contents

Introduction

Welcome to the "Complete Family Guide to Schizophrenia," a comprehensive resource designed to bridge the gap between clinical understanding and the day-to-day realities faced by families navigating the complexities of schizophrenia. This book is borne out of a profound respect for the resilience of individuals with schizophrenia and their families, and a recognition of the critical need for a holistic approach to support and care.

Schizophrenia is a condition that touches the lives of many, yet it remains enveloped in misconceptions and stigma. It is not merely a challenge for the individual diagnosed but also a profound life-changing reality for their families. As a mental health professional specializing in schizophrenia treatment and support, I have witnessed the incredible strength and dedication of families as they seek to provide love, understanding, and effective support to their loved ones. This guide is dedicated to you—the parents, siblings, partners, and children who stand by your loved ones on this journey.

Our journey through the pages of this book will begin with a foundational understanding of schizophrenia, exploring its causes, symptoms, and the latest research insights. This knowledge serves as the cornerstone of empathy and understanding, illuminating the experiences of your loved ones and guiding you towards more meaningful support and communication.

Recognizing the diverse needs and challenges faced by families, this guide will delve into practical strategies tailored to support both individuals with schizophrenia and their family members. From navigating the healthcare system and understanding treatment options to fostering a supportive home environment, we will cover a broad spectrum of topics relevant to your daily lives. The emphasis will be on promoting mental and emotional well-being for all family members, acknowledging that your health and resilience are paramount in the sustained support of your loved one.

Moreover, this book will explore the importance of effective communication within the family unit, offering tools and techniques to enhance understanding and empathy. By fostering open dialogue, we can break down barriers of fear and misunderstanding, creating a more inclusive and supportive family dynamic.

In addition to practical guidance, this book will also share stories of hope and resilience from families who have navigated the challenges of schizophrenia. These narratives serve as a testament to the strength of the human spirit and the power of love and support in the face of adversity.

Our goal is to empower you and your family with knowledge, understanding, and practical strategies to create a nurturing and supportive environment for your loved one with schizophrenia. Together, we can challenge the stigma surrounding mental health, celebrate progress, and embrace hope for a brighter future.

Thank you for embarking on this important journey with us. Your role in the life of your loved one with schizophrenia is invaluable, and through this guide, we hope to support, enlighten, and inspire you every step of the way.

Chapter 1: Understanding Schizophrenia

What is Schizophrenia?

Schizophrenia is a serious mental disorder characterized by a range of complex psychological symptoms. It affects a person's ability to think, feel, and behave clearly. The exact cause of schizophrenia isn't known, but a combination of genetics, brain chemistry, and environmental factors seems to play a role.

The symptoms of schizophrenia are often classified into three categories: positive, negative, and cognitive.

Positive symptoms are abnormal mental functions that are "added" to the person's personality. These include hallucinations (seeing or hearing things that aren't there), delusions (false beliefs), and thought disorders (unusual or dysfunctional ways of thinking).

1. **Hallucinations**: David, a 30-year-old with schizophrenia, commonly experiences auditory hallucinations. He hears voices commenting on his actions and constantly whispering negative thoughts, making it difficult for him to concentrate.

2. **Delusions**: Sarah, a 40-year-old diagnosed with schizophrenia, firmly believes that she has been chosen by a higher power to save the world from impending doom. She feels an overwhelming responsibility and is convinced of her special abilities that others don't understand.

3. **Disorganized Speech**: Michael, a 25-year-old with schizophrenia, often exhibits disorganized speech patterns. During conversations, his sentences may become incoherent or jump from one unrelated topic to another, making it challenging for others to follow his train of thought.

Negative symptoms are capabilities that are "lost" from the person's personality. These include reduced expression of emotions, reduced feelings of pleasure in everyday life, difficulty beginning and sustaining activities, and reduced speaking.

1. **Social Withdrawal**: Emily, a 35-year-old diagnosed with schizophrenia, gradually withdrew from her friends and family. She lost interest in social activities she used to enjoy and now prefers to isolate herself, leading to a lack of social interaction.

2. **Reduced Emotional Expression**: Maria, a 50-year-old with schizophrenia, displays limited facial expressions and vocal inflections. She often appears emotionally flat, showing reduced emotional responsiveness even in situations that would typically elicit strong emotions.

3. **Avolition**: John, a 28-year-old diagnosed with schizophrenia, struggles with avolition, which is the loss of motivation or ability to initiate and complete goal-directed activities. He finds it difficult to engage in basic self-care, pursue

employment opportunities, or even participate in hobbies he once enjoyed.

Cognitive symptoms affect the person's thought process. They can be subtle or severe and include trouble focusing or paying attention, poor executive functioning (the ability to understand information and use it to make decisions), and problems with working memory (the ability to use information immediately after learning it).

1. **Memory Impairment**: Lisa, a 45-year-old with schizophrenia, experiences significant memory problems, struggling to recall recent events and conversations. This impairment affects her ability to maintain a consistent daily routine and remember essential tasks or appointments.

2. **Attention Difficulties**: Chris, a 32-year-old diagnosed with schizophrenia, finds it hard to concentrate for extended periods. He frequently becomes easily distracted and has difficulty staying focused on tasks such as reading, studying, or engaging in conversations.

3. **Executive Dysfunction**: Susan, a 50-year-old with schizophrenia, experiences difficulties with executive functions, including planning, organizing, and decision-making. She often struggles to manage her daily responsibilities and may have trouble prioritizing tasks or setting goals.

The onset of schizophrenia symptoms typically occurs in late adolescence or early adulthood. Treatment is usually lifelong and often involves a combination of medications, psychotherapy, and coordinated specialty care services.

It's important to note that schizophrenia is not as common as other mental disorders, but the symptoms can be very disabling. Despite the challenges, many people with schizophrenia get better over time, not worse. With the right support and treatment, most people with schizophrenia can lead rewarding and meaningful lives.

Causes and Risk Factors

The exact causes of schizophrenia are not fully understood, but it's believed to be a combination of several factors, including genetics, brain chemistry and structure, and environmental factors.

1. Genetics:

Schizophrenia sometimes runs in families, suggesting that genes do play a role. However, it's important to note that just because someone in the family has schizophrenia, it doesn't mean other members will necessarily have it too. While the presence of certain genes may increase the risk, they don't cause the disorder by themselves.

2. Brain Chemistry and Structure:

People with schizophrenia often have differences in brain chemistry and structure. They usually have an imbalance in the chemical reactions involving neurotransmitters (substances that enable brain cells to communicate with each other) such as dopamine and glutamate.

Structural differences have also been observed in the brains of people with schizophrenia. However, these differences are not found in everyone with the disorder and could occur in individuals without the disorder too.

3. Environmental Factors:

Certain environmental factors seem to increase the risk of triggering schizophrenia in people who are genetically predisposed to the disorder. These can include exposure to viruses or malnutrition before birth, problems during birth, and psychosocial factors like stressful environmental conditions.

It's also worth mentioning that the use of psychoactive drugs during teen years and young adulthood has also been associated with the development of schizophrenia.

It's important to remember that while these factors can increase the risk, they don't guarantee that an individual will develop schizophrenia. The interaction of multiple genetic and environmental factors likely contribute to the onset of the disorder. This complex interplay is still a subject of ongoing research.

Types of Schizophrenia

Understanding schizophrenia can be a challenge, especially when it affects a loved one. Let's break it down into more simple terms, using the older classification system of subtypes for illustrative purposes.

it's important to understand that schizophrenia is not a monolithic condition. It manifests in different forms, each with its own unique set of symptoms and characteristics. Traditionally, there were five subtypes of schizophrenia: paranoid, disorganized, catatonic, undifferentiated, and residual. However, the most recent edition of the Diagnostic and Statistical Manual of Mental Disorders (DSM-5) no longer uses these subtypes. Instead, it classifies schizophrenia based on the severity and presence of key symptoms such as delusions, hallucinations, and disorganized speech.

Despite this change, the traditional subtypes can still provide useful insights into the diverse manifestations of schizophrenia. Let's dive deeper:

1. **Paranoid Schizophrenia:** This was the most common subtype of schizophrenia. People with this form primarily have positive symptoms such as delusions and hallucinations. For instance, an individual might believe they're being followed or persecuted without any evidence. These delusions can often lead to high levels of anxiety and fear.

Case Study: John, a 30-year old man, began to believe that his neighbors were spying on him and planning to harm him. Despite reassurances from family and friends, he remained convinced of this perceived threat, leading to significant distress and social withdrawal.

2. **Disorganized Schizophrenia:** In this subtype, individuals typically exhibit disorganized thinking, speech, and behavior, along with negative symptoms like emotional flatness. Their speech

might be hard to follow, and their behavior could be bizarre or purposeless.

Case Study: Emily, a 25-year old woman, started speaking in a way that was difficult for others to understand, often switching topics abruptly or giving answers unrelated to the questions asked. She also displayed inappropriate emotional responses, like laughing in a serious situation.

3. **Catatonic Schizophrenia:** This rare subtype is characterized by periods of immobility or excessive, purposeless movement. Individuals might also mimic others' speech or movement, a symptom known as echolalia or echopraxia.

Case Study: Mark, a 27-year old man, was found in a park maintaining a rigid posture and staring into the distance for hours. At other times, he would suddenly start running around aimlessly.

4. **Undifferentiated Schizophrenia:** This subtype was diagnosed when an individual had symptoms of schizophrenia but did not meet the specific criteria for the paranoid, disorganized, or catatonic subtypes.

5. **Residual Schizophrenia:** This subtype was used for individuals who had a history of schizophrenia, but were not currently showing prominent symptoms. They might still have some negative symptoms or less severe positive symptoms.

Case Study: Sarah, a 35-year old woman with a history of schizophrenia, was no longer experiencing hallucinations or delusions. However, she still struggled with a lack of motivation and emotional flatness, which affected her ability to maintain daily activities.

Please remember that these subtypes are now considered outdated, but they can still offer a useful framework for understanding the varied presentations of schizophrenia. Today, a diagnosis of schizophrenia involves a thorough evaluation of symptoms, their duration, and the impact on the individual's ability to function.

Diagnosing Schizophrenia

Diagnosing schizophrenia isn't always easy. Doctors usually follow these steps:

1. **Physical Exam:** This may be done to help rule out other problems that could be causing symptoms and to check for any related complications.

2. **Psychiatric Evaluation:** This includes observing the person's appearance and demeanor, asking about thoughts, moods, hallucinations, delusions, substance use, and potentially violence or suicidal thoughts. It can also include a discussion of family and personal history.

3. **Diagnostic Criteria for Schizophrenia:** For a diagnosis of schizophrenia, some symptoms must be present for at least six months with at least one month of active symptoms.

4. **Medical History and Exams:** Tests and screenings may be conducted to rule out other conditions and to check for alcohol and drugs. The doctor might

also request imaging studies, such as an MRI or CT scan.

5. **Psychological Assessment:** A psychologist may also assess the person's mental state by observing appearance and demeanor and asking about thoughts, moods, delusions, hallucinations, substance use, and the potential for violence or suicide.

Comorbidities Associated with Schizophrenia

People with schizophrenia often have additional (comorbid) mental health disorders including:

- Substance use disorders

- Anxiety disorders

- Depression

- Obsessive-compulsive disorder (OCD)

Doctors would usually use similar methods as above to diagnose these conditions, such as personal evaluation, medical history, and psychological assessments.

Understanding the primary clinical symptoms of schizophrenia and behavioral patterns exhibited by patients is essential for early diagnosis and appropriate treatment. Healthcare providers use various diagnostic tools, including self-reported symptoms, personal evaluation, medical history and exams, and psychological assessments, to screen and diagnose this disorder. Additionally, they assess for comorbidities such as substance abuse, anxiety disorders, mood disorders, OCD, and PTSD to provide a comprehensive diagnosis. Remember, seeking professional help is crucial for accurate diagnosis and effective management of schizophrenia and its associated conditions.

Chapter 2: Living with Schizophrenia 1

The Lived Experience

Living with schizophrenia is a unique journey that can be challenging due to the symptoms it entails. These symptoms include hallucinations, delusions, thought disorder, and negative symptoms like apathy or lack of motivation. The experience of living with schizophrenia varies widely between individuals, with some finding it debilitating, while others manage to lead fulfilling lives with the right treatment and support.

Family support plays a crucial role in the lives of individuals living with schizophrenia. A supportive family can provide emotional help, assist with daily tasks, and help navigate the healthcare system.

Families often need to learn about the illness to provide effective support. This can include understanding the symptoms of schizophrenia, knowing how to respond during a crisis, and being aware of the resources available for help.

Being a caregiver can also be challenging. It's important for family members to take care of their own mental health and seek support when needed. Support groups and counseling can provide a space to share experiences, learn from others, and find comfort in knowing they're not alone

Stigma and Misconceptions

Stigma is one of the most significant challenges faced by people living with schizophrenia. They often encounter misconceptions and stereotypes that can exacerbate their condition. It is important to address these issues and promote understanding to create a more inclusive and supportive society. Let's explore stigma and misconceptions related to schizophrenia.

Stigma:

a) Social Stereotypes: Stigma arises from widely held beliefs and stereotypes about mental health conditions, including schizophrenia. These stereotypes often portray individuals with schizophrenia as dangerous, unpredictable, or incapable of leading fulfilling lives. Such perceptions contribute to fear, discrimination, and social exclusion.

b) Discrimination: Stigmatization may result in discriminatory practices, such as limited employment opportunities, housing challenges, or limited access to healthcare. This further exacerbates the obstacles faced by individuals with schizophrenia, affecting their overall well-being and quality of life.

c) Self-Stigma: Stigma can also lead to self-stigma, wherein individuals internalize negative beliefs and attitudes about their condition. Self-stigma can lower self-esteem, hinder help-seeking behaviors, and hinder individuals from fully participating in society.

Misconceptions:

a) Violence and Schizophrenia: One common misconception is the association between schizophrenia and violence. While it is true that individuals with untreated or uncontrolled symptoms may experience distress and exhibit challenging behaviors, the majority of individuals with schizophrenia are not violent. In reality, they are more likely to be victims of violence rather than perpetrators.

b) Split Personality: Another misconception is the belief that schizophrenia involves a split personality or multiple personalities. Schizophrenia is a distinct mental disorder characterized by a disruption in thoughts, perceptions, and emotions. It is important to differentiate it from dissociative identity disorder (formerly known as multiple personality disorder), which is a separate condition.

c) Hopelessness and Recovery: There is a widespread misconception that individuals with schizophrenia cannot recover or lead fulfilling lives. With early intervention, appropriate treatment, support systems, and personal resilience, many individuals with schizophrenia can manage symptoms, pursue meaningful activities, and achieve personal goals.

d) Intelligence and Schizophrenia: Contrary to popular belief, intelligence is not a determining factor in the development of schizophrenia. Schizophrenia can affect individuals from all walks of life, regardless of their intellectual abilities or achievements.

Addressing Stigma and Misconceptions:

a) Education and Awareness: Education plays a vital role in addressing stigma and misconceptions surrounding schizophrenia. Increasing public awareness about the condition, sharing accurate information, and challenging stereotypes can help break down barriers and foster understanding.

b) Personal Stories and Lived Experience Personal Stories and Lived Experience: Sharing personal stories and experiences of individuals with schizophrenia can humanize the condition and create empathy. Hearing firsthand accounts can challenge stereotypes and misconceptions, illustrating that individuals with schizophrenia are unique individuals with their own desires, talents, and aspirations.

c) Language Matters: Using respectful and person-centered language is crucial when discussing schizophrenia. Avoiding derogatory terms and using language that promotes dignity and respect can help reduce stigma and create a more inclusive environment.

d) Media Representation: Accurate and responsible representation of schizophrenia in the media is essential. Encouraging media outlets to portray realistic and nuanced depictions of individuals with schizophrenia can aid in dispelling myths and fostering understanding.

e) Support and Empathy: Providing support and empathy to individuals with schizophrenia and their families is vital. Creating a compassionate and non-judgmental environment can help alleviate some of the stigma and support their journey towards recovery and well-being.

How families can support against stigma and misconceptions

Families play a pivotal role in supporting their loved ones against the stigma and misconceptions associated with mental health conditions, such as schizophrenia. Here are some strategies families can adopt:

1. Psychoeducation: Families can benefit from learning about their loved one's mental health condition. This education can help to dispel myths and misconceptions about mental illness, allowing family members to better empathize with the patient and avoid unintentional stigmatizing behaviors.

2. Personal Contact and Sharing Experiences: Research shows that knowing or having contact with someone with a mental illness is one of the best ways to reduce stigma. For families, this means sharing their experiences and encouraging open discussions about mental health.

3. Speaking Out Against Stigma: Families can take an active role in challenging stigma by expressing their opinions at events, in letters to the editor, or on the internet. Speaking out can help instill courage in others facing similar challenges and contribute to broader societal change.

4. Education and Responding to Misperceptions: Families can help reduce stigma by educating themselves and others about mental health. Responding to misperceptions or negative comments with accurate information can help to challenge harmful stereotypes.

5. Focusing on the Positive: Rather than focusing solely on the challenges of mental illness, families can highlight the strengths and abilities of their loved ones. This can help to challenge the misconception that people with mental illness are defined by their condition.

6. Advocacy: Families can engage in advocacy work to help break down mental health stigma. This could involve supporting organizations that promote mental health awareness, or advocating for policies that support individuals with mental health conditions.

While the stigma surrounding mental health conditions can be a significant barrier, families can play a crucial role in combating this stigma. By educating themselves and others, speaking out against stigma, and advocating for their loved ones, families can help to create a more understanding and compassionate society.

Impact on the Individual and Family

Schizophrenia can significantly impact an individual's life. It can affect their ability to study, work, maintain relationships, and carry out daily tasks. This impact extends to the family as well, with many family members becoming caregivers and experiencing significant stress and emotional burden.Understanding this impact is crucial for providing support and navigating the challenges that may arise. Let's explore the effects of a schizophrenia diagnosis on the individual and their family.

Impact on the Individual:

a) Emotional Distress: Receiving a diagnosis of schizophrenia can evoke a wide range of emotions, including fear, confusion, sadness, and anxiety. The individual may struggle with accepting and understanding their condition, as well as coping with the implications it has for their life.

b) Disrupted Life Plans: Schizophrenia often disrupts an individual's life plans and aspirations. This can include challenges in pursuing education, maintaining employment, or engaging in social activities. Adjusting to these changes may be difficult and require additional support.

c) Medication Management: Treatment for schizophrenia frequently involves medication management. Adapting to a new medication regimen and dealing with potential side effects can be challenging for the individual. Consistency with medication is essential for managing symptoms effectively.

d) Social Relationships: Schizophrenia can significantly impact an individual's social interactions and relationships. Symptoms such as disorganized thinking, social withdrawal, and difficulties in communication can isolate the individual and affect their ability to engage in meaningful connections with others.

e) Self-Stigma: Individuals diagnosed with schizophrenia may experience self-stigma, internalizing the negative stereotypes and misconceptions associated with the condition. This can lead to lowered self-esteem, reduced self-confidence, and feelings of shame or inadequacy.

Impact on the Family:

a) Emotional Challenges: Family members often experience a range of emotional challenges when a loved one is diagnosed with schizophrenia. They may feel worried, overwhelmed, frustrated, and even guilty for not being able to fully understand or help their loved one.

b) Changed Family Dynamics: The presence of schizophrenia may alter family dynamics, leading to increased stress and tension. Roles and responsibilities within the family may shift to accommodate the needs of the individual with schizophrenia, which can impact the relationships between family members.

c) Support and Caregiving: Family members often become primary caregivers for individuals with schizophrenia. This responsibility can be demanding, both physically and emotionally. It may involve monitoring medication, accompanying the individual to appointments, providing emotional support, and engaging in crisis management.

d) Financial Strain: Managing the financial aspects of schizophrenia, including medical expenses, therapy sessions, and prescription medications, can create a financial burden for the individual and their family. This additional stress may contribute to overall family strain.

e) Community Education and Advocacy: Families may become advocates for their loved one and the broader community. They may engage in educating others about schizophrenia to reduce stigma, promote understanding, and advocate for better resources and support for individuals with schizophrenia.

The diagnosis of schizophrenia can have a significant impact on both the individual diagnosed and their family. Emotional distress, disrupted life plans, medication management, changes in social relationships, and self-stigma are some of the challenges faced by individuals living with schizophrenia. Family members may experience emotional challenges, changes in family dynamics, increased caregiving responsibilities, financial strain, and may become advocates for their loved one and the community. It is crucial for individuals and families to have access to appropriate support, including mental health services, education, and resources, to navigate the impact of schizophrenia on their lives. With understanding, empathy, and a supportive network, individuals and families can work towards managing the condition and improving overall well-being.

In conclusion, living with schizophrenia is a complex experience marked by numerous challenges. However, with the right support and understanding, individuals with schizophrenia can lead fulfilling lives, and their families can navigate this journey alongside them.

Families Shared Experience
Here are three real-life examples of families dealing with a loved one diagnosed with schizophrenia, each illustrating different aspects of the impact this condition can have:

1. The Smith Family

In the Smith family, their eldest son, John, was diagnosed with schizophrenia during his first year at university. The initial shock and confusion were overwhelming. They didn't understand why their bright, outgoing son had suddenly become withdrawn and was hearing voices that weren't there.

The emotional impact was significant. They felt a deep sense of grief for the life they thought John would have, now replaced with uncertainty and fear about what the future held. They also struggled with feelings of guilt, wondering if they could have done something to prevent it.

As John's condition worsened, his parents had to take on the role of caregivers. They juggled managing his medications, attending doctor's appointments, and dealing with episodes of acute psychosis. This increased responsibility put a strain on their own mental health and their relationship.

Despite these challenges, the Smiths sought help from mental health professionals who provided them with support and resources. They also joined a local support group for families affected by schizophrenia, which provided a platform to share their experiences and learn from others in similar situations.

2. The Garcia Family

For the Garcias, their daughter Maria's diagnosis came when she was just starting her career. Maria had been living independently, but as her symptoms worsened, she had to move back home. This brought about significant financial strain as the family had to shoulder the costs of treatment and care.

The Garcias faced stigma and discrimination from their community, leading to social isolation. Friends stopped visiting, and extended family members kept their distance, unsure of how to interact with Maria.

However, the Garcias found strength in each other. They educated themselves about schizophrenia, learning how to best support Maria while also taking care of their own mental health. They became advocates in their community, challenging misconceptions about mental health and working towards reducing the stigma associated with it.

3. The Patel Family

The Patels had a different journey. Their mother, Sunita, was diagnosed with schizophrenia later in life. This shifted the family dynamics significantly as the children, now adults, had to step into caregiving roles for their mother.

Balancing their own careers and families while caring for their mother was challenging. They also had to navigate the healthcare system, advocating for their mother's needs and ensuring she received the appropriate care.

The Patels found solace in online support groups and forums, where they could connect with others dealing with similar situations. They learned about resources available for caregivers and strategies to manage the stress associated with caregiving.

In each of these examples, the families faced significant challenges due to their loved one's diagnosis of schizophrenia. However, they also demonstrated resilience, seeking help, educating themselves, and finding ways to cope with the emotional, financial, and social impacts.

Chapter 3: Treatment Options

Medical Treatments

Schizophrenia is a complex mental health disorder, but recent advances in treatment options provide hope for patients and their families. This guide aims to explore some of the latest groundbreaking treatments, comparing them with traditional methods and discussing their benefits, risks, side effects, cost, and availability.

New Treatments

1. Glia-Targeted Treatments

Recent research has highlighted the role of glial cells - non-neuronal brain cells - in psychiatric conditions like schizophrenia. New treatments targeting these cells aim to correct the diseased and damaged glia, potentially revolutionizing the field of psychiatry.

Benefits: These treatments could potentially address the root cause of schizophrenia, rather than just managing symptoms.

Risks & Side Effects: As this is a relatively new area of research, the risks and side effects are not yet fully understood.

Cost & Availability: These treatments are still in the research phase and are not yet commercially available.

2. Pharmacogenetics

Pharmacogenetics involves tailoring antipsychotic drug therapy to the individual's genetic makeup. This personalized approach could drastically improve treatment effectiveness and reduce side effects.

Benefits: Increased effectiveness of drugs, reduced side effects, and potentially faster recovery times.

Risks & Side Effects: Genetic testing raises privacy concerns, and not all patients will benefit from pharmacogenetic treatment.

Cost & Availability: While genetic testing is becoming more accessible, it can be expensive and may not be covered by all insurance plans.

Traditional Treatments

1.Antipsychotic Medications

These are usually the first line of treatment for schizophrenia. They work by altering the brain's chemical balance to help manage symptoms.

Benefits: Antipsychotics can significantly reduce symptoms, such as hallucinations, delusions, and disorganized thinking, leading to improved quality of life.

Risks & Side Effects: Common side effects include drowsiness, dizziness, weight gain, and movement problems. In rare cases, long-term use may lead to a condition called tardive dyskinesia, which involves involuntary movements.

Cost & Availability: Costs can vary widely based on insurance coverage and whether a generic version is available. These medications are widely available through prescription.

2.Psychotherapy

Psychotherapy, or "talk therapy", can be very effective when combined with medication. Cognitive-behavioral therapy (CBT) and family therapy are commonly used.

Benefits: Psychotherapy can help patients better understand their condition, manage symptoms, address challenges, and improve communication and relationships.

Risks & Side Effects: There are few risks associated with psychotherapy. However, it requires commitment and can bring up uncomfortable emotions.

Cost & Availability: The cost of therapy sessions can vary greatly depending on location, insurance coverage, and whether the therapist operates on a sliding scale. Many therapists offer virtual sessions, increasing accessibility.

2.Electroconvulsive Therapy (ECT)

ECT is typically reserved for cases where other treatments haven't worked. It involves sending small electric currents through the brain to trigger a brief seizure.

Benefits: ECT can provide rapid relief of severe symptoms and is especially effective for treating catatonic schizophrenia.

Risks & Side Effects: ECT can cause side effects like temporary memory loss, confusion, and physical risks associated with anesthesia.

Cost & Availability: ECT is more expensive than other treatments and is typically used as a last resort. It's available in most major hospitals.

Coordinated Specialty Care (CSC)

CSC is a team approach that combines medication, psychotherapy, family involvement, case management, and work or education support.

Benefits: CSC has been shown to be particularly beneficial for individuals who are experiencing their first episode of psychosis.

Risks & Side Effects: There are few risks associated with CSC. However, it requires a significant commitment from the patient and their family.

Cost & Availability: The cost can be higher due to the comprehensive nature of the program. Availability varies by region, but it's becoming increasingly common.

Comparison with Traditional Treatments

Traditional treatments for schizophrenia typically involve a combination of antipsychotic medications and psychotherapy. While these treatments can be effective, they often come with side effects such as weight gain, drowsiness, and movement disorders. In comparison, the new treatments discussed above aim to reduce these side effects and improve treatment effectiveness.

Upcoming Treatments

Research into new therapies for schizophrenia is ongoing. One promising area is the use of deep brain stimulation, a surgical procedure that has been successful in treating conditions like Parkinson's disease.

Supporting Information

Clinical trials and research studies are crucial for advancing our understanding of schizophrenia and developing new treatments. To stay up-to-date on the latest research, families can visit clinical trial databases like ClinicalTrials.gov.

Complementary Therapies & Lifestyle Changes

In addition to medical treatment, lifestyle changes and complementary therapies can support recovery. This could include regular physical activity, a balanced diet, adequate sleep, stress management techniques, and joining support groups.

Remember, every individual's experience with schizophrenia is unique. What works best will depend on the specific symptoms, overall health, and personal preferences. It's crucial to have open and ongoing conversations with healthcare providers to ensure the treatment plan meets the individual's needs and promotes the best possible outcome.While this guide provides an overview of the latest treatments, it's crucial to consult with a healthcare provider before making any changes to a treatment plan.

Therapeutic Interventions
Cognitive Behavioral Therapy (CBT)

Cognitive Behavioral Therapy (CBT) is a widely used intervention for individuals with schizophrenia. It is a type of psychotherapy that focuses on helping individuals with schizophrenia identify and change negative thought patterns and behaviors that contribute to distressing symptoms.

Here is a brief explanation of the CBT intervention for schizophrenia:

1. Psychoeducation: The first step in CBT for schizophrenia is providing psychoeducation about the illness. This involves educating the individual and their family about the symptoms, causes, and course of the disorder. It helps to reduce stigma, enhance understanding, and encourage active participation in treatment.

2. Collaboration and Goal Setting: Therapists work collaboratively with individuals with schizophrenia

to set treatment goals. These goals can include reducing symptoms, improving functioning, enhancing coping skills, and promoting overall well-being.

3. Cognitive Restructuring: CBT focuses on identifying and challenging distorted or irrational thoughts and beliefs that contribute to distressing symptoms. The therapist helps the individual examine the evidence for and against these thoughts, and develop more balanced and realistic alternatives. For example, if someone with schizophrenia believes that others are constantly judging them, the therapist helps them explore alternative explanations and develop more adaptive thoughts.

4. Behavioral Techniques: CBT for schizophrenia incorporates various behavioral techniques to address problematic behaviors. These may include activity scheduling, where individuals are encouraged to engage in structured and pleasurable activities, as well as social skills training to improve interpersonal interactions and reduce social isolation.

5. Reality Testing: Schizophrenia is often characterized by perceptual distortions (hallucinations) and fixed false beliefs (delusions). In CBT, reality testing techniques are used to help individuals evaluate the accuracy of their experiences. They learn to gather evidence and consider alternative explanations for their beliefs,

thereby challenging and modifying their distorted perceptions.

6. Coping Strategies: CBT helps individuals develop effective coping strategies to manage symptoms and stressors associated with schizophrenia. These strategies may include relaxation techniques, problem-solving skills, and stress management.

7. Relapse Prevention: CBT aims to equip individuals with schizophrenia with skills to prevent relapse and maintain recovery. Strategies such as identifying early warning signs, implementing coping strategies, and developing a relapse prevention plan are important components of CBT.

It is worth noting that CBT for schizophrenia is typically delivered in combination with medication management and other psychosocial interventions. The specific techniques and strategies used may vary based on the individual's needs and treatment goals.

Benefits: CBT can help manage symptoms, reduce the frequency and intensity of psychotic episodes, and improve overall quality of life.

Risks & Side Effects: There are minimal risks associated with CBT. Some people might initially find it uncomfortable discussing personal thoughts and feelings.

Cost & Availability: The cost can vary depending on the therapist and location. Many therapists now offer online sessions, making it more accessible.

Family Therapy

Family Therapy is an essential intervention for individuals with schizophrenia as it recognizes the significance of involving the family in the treatment process. It aims to improve communication, reduce stress, enhance problem-solving skills, and promote the overall well-being of both the individual with schizophrenia and their family members.

Here is a detailed explanation of Family Therapy for schizophrenia:

1. Education and Psychoeducation: Family Therapy begins by providing education and psychoeducation about schizophrenia to the family members. This includes information about symptoms, causes, and treatment options. It helps the family understand the impact of the illness on their loved one and the family dynamics.

2. Communication and Expressing Emotions: Family Therapy focuses on improving communication skills within the family. It encourages open dialogue and provides a safe space for family members to express their emotions and concerns about schizophrenia. Effective communication reduces misunderstandings, conflicts, and fosters better support for the individual with schizophrenia.

3. Reducing Expressed Emotion: Expressed emotion refers to the family's critical, hostile, or emotionally over-involved attitudes towards the individual with schizophrenia. Family Therapy aims to reduce

expressed emotion as it has been linked to higher relapse rates and poorer outcomes. By promoting empathy, understanding, and support, the therapy helps create a more nurturing and supportive family environment.

4. Problem-Solving and Coping Skills: Family Therapy helps family members develop problem-solving and coping skills to deal with the challenges associated with schizophrenia. It encourages the development of effective strategies for managing symptoms, handling stress, and enhancing daily functioning.

5. Enhancing Social Support: The therapy emphasizes the importance of social support for individuals with schizophrenia. Family members are encouraged to provide emotional and practical support, facilitate social activities, and facilitate community integration. This helps reduce social isolation and promotes the individual's overall well-being.

6. Managing Relapse and Crisis Prevention: Family Therapy provides strategies for identifying early signs of relapse or crisis and developing a plan to manage such situations. This involves recognizing warning signs, establishing communication channels, and implementing strategies to prevent or minimize the impact of relapse.

7. Family Psychoeducation and Support: Families are provided with ongoing psychoeducation and

support throughout the treatment process. Education about schizophrenia, coping strategies, and available resources helps families become better equipped to support their loved ones. In addition, support groups and resources may be offered for families to connect with others facing similar challenges.

Family Therapy for schizophrenia is typically delivered by a licensed mental health professional, such as a psychologist or a licensed marriage and family therapist. The number of sessions and specific techniques used may vary based during on the treatment required.

Benefits: Family therapy can reduce stress within the home, provide family members with a better understanding of schizophrenia, and equip them with strategies to support their loved one.

Risks & Side Effects: Family therapy requires commitment from all participants, which can sometimes be challenging to coordinate. It may also bring up sensitive family issues.

Cost & Availability: The cost of family therapy varies greatly. Many therapists offer sliding scale fees based on income. It's widely available in-person or via teletherapy.

Art Therapy

Art therapy uses creative activities as a form of expression. It can be a useful tool for those who find it difficult to express their feelings verbally.

Benefits: Art therapy offers a safe and creative outlet for emotions. It can help reduce anxiety, increase self-esteem, and improve mood.

Risks & Side Effects: There are very few risks associated with art therapy. However, it might not be suitable for everyone.

Cost & Availability: The cost can vary. Some community centers offer free or low-cost art therapy sessions. It's becoming increasingly available in mental health clinics and hospitals.

Social Skills Training

Social Skills Training (SST) is an intervention technique used in the treatment of schizophrenia to help individuals develop and improve their social skills and interpersonal interactions. It aims to address the social deficits often associated with schizophrenia and enhance the individual's ability to engage in meaningful social relationships. Here is a detailed explanation of Social Skills Training for schizophrenia:

1. Assessment: The first step in SST is to assess the individual's current social functioning and identify specific areas where improvement is needed. This may involve evaluating their communication skills, social interactions, problem-solving abilities, and the impact of symptoms on social functioning.

2. Psychoeducation: Psychoeducation about social skills and the importance of social interactions is provided to the individual. They learn about the

specific social deficits associated with schizophrenia and how these deficits can impact their daily life and relationships.

3. Skill Identification: The therapist works with the individual to identify specific social skills that need to be developed or improved upon. These may include communication skills (verbal and non-verbal), active listening, assertiveness, conflict resolution, empathy, and social problem-solving skills.

4. Modeling: The therapist demonstrates the targeted social skills to the individual, providing them with an observation of how specific skills are performed. This helps the individual understand the desired behaviors and provides a visual model for learning.

5. Behavioral Rehearsal: The individual is given opportunities to practice the identified social skills in a safe and supportive environment. Role-playing exercises or simulated social situations are used to simulate real-life scenarios, allowing the individual to practice appropriate responses and behaviors.

6. Feedback and Reinforcement: During the practice sessions, the therapist provides constructive feedback, highlighting areas of improvement and reinforcing positive behaviors. Positive reinforcement, such as praise or rewards, is used to encourage and motivate the individual.

7. Generalization: SST focuses on helping the individual generalize the learned social skills to

real-life situations. This involves practicing the skills in various settings, such as at home, work, or social gatherings. The individual is encouraged to apply the skills outside of therapy sessions and to seek social opportunities to further practice and develop their skills.

8. Coping Strategies: SST also includes teaching the individual coping strategies to manage social anxiety or other symptoms that may hinder social interactions. Techniques such as relaxation exercises and cognitive restructuring are incorporated to help the individual manage anxiety-provoking social situations.

9. Maintenance and Follow-up: SST is an ongoing process, and regular follow-up sessions are conducted to support the individual's progress and address any new challenges that may arise.

Benefits: Improving these skills can lead to increased independence, better interpersonal relationships, and improved quality of life.

Risks & Side Effects: There are minimal risks associated with social skills training. However, it requires ongoing practice to maintain and improve these skills.

Cost & Availability: Costs can vary, but some community mental health programs offer free or low-cost training. It's widely available in mental health clinics and rehabilitation centers.

Remember, each person's journey with schizophrenia is unique. The best therapeutic interventions depend on the individual's symptoms, lifestyle, and personal preferences. Open communication with healthcare providers is crucial to ensure the treatment plan meets the individual's needs and promotes the best possible outcome.

Detailed Insights on Schizophrenia Treatment

Schizophrenia is a complex condition, and understanding its treatment can be challenging. Here are three real-life scenarios of individuals navigating their journey with schizophrenia, including how they managed the side effects of their medications.

Medication Management: Alice's Journey

Alice, a 30-year-old woman, started to hear voices that others couldn't perceive. She was diagnosed with schizophrenia following a psychiatric assessment.

Symptoms: Auditory hallucinations, paranoia, and social withdrawal were among Alice's main symptoms.

Treatment and Side Effects Management: Alice was prescribed haloperidol, an antipsychotic medication. This medication significantly reduced her hallucinations and paranoia, enhancing her overall quality of life. However, side effects such as drowsiness, difficulty sleeping, and restlessness were potential issues. Alice managed these by adjusting her medication timings under her doctor's guidance, ensuring she took her medication at times when the side effects would least interfere with her daily activities.

Cost: The cost of medication can vary widely, depending on insurance coverage and location.

Outcome: With regular medication and check-ups, Alice saw a significant reduction in her symptoms. She returned to work and reconnected with her loved ones.

2. Combination Therapy: Ben's Path

Ben, a 22-year-old college student, began experiencing delusions, disorganized speech, and lack of motivation. He was eventually diagnosed with schizophrenia.

Symptoms: Delusions, disorganized thinking, and a marked decrease in his overall function were among Ben's symptoms.

Treatment and Side Effects Management: Ben's treatment involved a combination of loxapine, an antipsychotic medication, and cognitive-behavioral therapy (CBT). While the medication and therapy helped Ben manage his symptoms and improve his social relationships, he did experience side effects such as dizziness and drowsiness from the medication. Ben dealt with these by scheduling activities requiring concentration at times when the medication's effects were minimal.

Cost: The cost of therapy can vary greatly, depending on the therapist, location, and insurance coverage.

Outcome: With consistent therapy and medication, Ben returned to his studies.

3. Comprehensive Approach: Clara's Experience

Clara, a 27-year-old woman, had been living with schizophrenia for several years. Her symptoms were poorly controlled, leading to frequent hospitalizations.

Symptoms: Clara experienced severe hallucinations, delusions, and social withdrawal.

Treatment and Side Effects Management: Clara's treatment plan included chlorpromazine, an antipsychotic medication, family therapy, and a focus on honing her socialization skills. Though the comprehensive approach helped stabilize Clara's condition, side effects like dizziness and blurred vision from the medication were issues. Clara managed these by taking her medication at bedtime and using prescription glasses to help with her vision.

Cost: Family therapy costs vary significantly, depending on the therapist and location. Some therapists offer sliding scale fees based on income.

Outcome: With her family's support and the healthcare team's assistance, Clara maintained more consistent wellness.

These stories highlight the various treatment approaches for schizophrenia, reflecting each individual's unique experience. They underscore the importance of personalized treatment plans, consistent follow-up, and loved ones' support in managing schizophrenia.

The Role of Lifestyle Changes

The role of lifestyle changes in the management of schizophrenia is increasingly recognized as an important aspect of treatment. While medication and therapy are typically the primary interventions, adopting healthy lifestyle habits can significantly contribute to overall well-being, symptom management, and recovery for individuals with schizophrenia. Here are several lifestyle changes that can play a beneficial role:

1. Physical Activity: Regular exercise has been shown to have positive effects on both physical and mental health. It can help reduce symptoms of schizophrenia, improve mood, increase energy levels, enhance cognitive function, and promote overall well-being. Engaging in activities such as walking, jogging, swimming, or yoga can be beneficial.

2. Balanced Diet: A nutritious and well-balanced diet can support brain health and enhance overall physical health. Consuming a variety of fruits, vegetables, whole grains, lean proteins, and healthy fats can provide essential nutrients and contribute to better overall well-being. It is important to consult with a healthcare professional or nutritionist to optimize dietary choices.

3. Adequate Sleep: Getting sufficient and quality sleep is essential for mental health. Sleep disturbances are common in individuals with schizophrenia and can exacerbate symptoms. Developing healthy sleep habits and practicing good sleep hygiene, such as maintaining a regular sleep schedule, creating a calming bedtime routine, and creating a comfortable sleep environment, can improve sleep quality.

4. Avoiding Substance Abuse: Substance abuse, including alcohol and illicit drugs, can significantly worsen symptoms and interfere with treatment outcomes for individuals with schizophrenia. It is important to avoid or minimize substance use to promote better mental health and reduce the risk of relapse.

5. Stress Management: Effective stress management techniques can help reduce symptom severity and improve overall well-being. Strategies such as mindfulness meditation, deep breathing exercises, relaxation techniques, and engaging in hobbies or activities that promote relaxation and enjoyment can help individuals cope with stress more effectively.

6. Social Support: Maintaining a strong support system and engaging in social activities can contribute to better mental health outcomes. Socializing with family, friends, and peer support groups can provide emotional support, reduce feelings of isolation, and promote a sense of belonging.

7. Maintaining Routine: Establishing and maintaining a structured daily routine can be helpful for individuals with schizophrenia. Having a predictable schedule for activities such as waking up, meal times, medication, therapy sessions, and leisure activities can provide a sense of stability and reduce stress.

8. Managing Co-occurring Health Conditions: Individuals with schizophrenia often have increased risk for physical health conditions such as obesity, diabetes, and cardiovascular disease. Managing these conditions through regular screenings, appropriate medication use, and lifestyle modifications can help improve overall health outcomes and contribute to long-term well-being.

It is important to note that lifestyle changes should be integrated into a comprehensive treatment plan for schizophrenia, in collaboration with healthcare professionals. These changes should not replace medication or therapy but rather be seen as complementary strategies to enhance overall wellness.

Adopting and sustaining healthy lifestyle habits can require motivation, support, and guidance. Healthcare professionals, including psychiatrists, therapists, and other members of the treatment team, can provide education, resources, and support in implementing and maintaining these lifestyle changes. Additionally, family members and caregivers can play a significant role in supporting and encouraging individuals with schizophrenia in their journey towards a healthier lifestyle.

Family's Role in Supporting Lifestyle Changes

The family plays a crucial role in supporting lifestyle changes for individuals with schizophrenia. Their involvement, encouragement, and understanding can greatly contribute to the success and long-term sustainability of these changes. Here are ways in which the family can support lifestyle changes:

1. Education and Awareness: Family members can educate themselves about schizophrenia and the importance of lifestyle changes in the management of the condition. Understanding the benefits of healthy habits can help them provide informed support to their loved one.

2. Encouragement and Motivation: Family members can offer words of encouragement and support to help their loved one stay motivated and committed to making positive lifestyle changes. Expressing belief in their ability to make and sustain these changes can make a significant difference.

3. Setting a Healthy Example: Modeling healthy behaviors within the family can be an effective way to promote lifestyle changes. When family members adopt healthy habits themselves, such as engaging in regular physical activity or maintaining a balanced diet, it sends a positive message and can inspire the individual with schizophrenia to do the same.

4. Collaboration in Meal Planning: Involving the individual in meal planning and preparation can be a collaborative effort within the family. Encouraging nutritious food choices and preparing meals together can make the experience more enjoyable and increase the chances of successful dietary changes.

5. Active Participation in Physical Activity: Encouraging and participating in physical activities with the individual can make exercising more enjoyable and motivate them to engage in regular physical activity. Family members can join in activities such as walks, sporting activities, or even workout sessions together.

6. Creating a Supportive Environment: Family members can create an environment that promotes and supports healthy habits. This can include minimizing the presence of unhealthy foods in the household, providing encouragement and reminders for medication adherence, and creating a calm and structured atmosphere that supports adequate sleep.

7. Supporting Stress Management: Stress can negatively impact lifestyle changes and overall well-being. Family members can assist in identifying stressors and supporting the individual in implementing stress management techniques such as engaging in relaxation exercises or participating in stress-reducing activities together.

8. Communication and Collaboration with Treatment Team: The family can actively participate in treatment planning and collaborate with the individual's healthcare professionals. This involves attending therapy sessions, providing relevant information to the treatment team, and maintaining open lines of communication to ensure a comprehensive approach to care.

9. Patience and Understanding: Lifestyle changes can be challenging, and individuals with schizophrenia may experience setbacks or difficulty maintaining consistent habits. Providing understanding, patience, and support during these times can be instrumental in helping them continue their efforts towards living a healthy lifestyle .

10. Creating a Support Network: In addition to family support, individuals with schizophrenia can benefit from connecting with support networks such as support groups, community organizations, and peer groups. Family members can help their loved ones find and access these resources, which can provide additional encouragement, guidance, and a sense of belonging.

11. Monitoring and Accountability: Family members can play a role in monitoring progress and providing accountability for lifestyle changes. This can involve tracking medication adherence, joining in on exercise routines, or offering reminders for healthy habits. This gentle support can help individuals stay on track and maintain focus.

12. Celebrating Achievements and Milestones: Recognizing and celebrating achievements, no matter how small, can boost motivation and reinforce the positive impact of lifestyle changes. Family members can acknowledge and celebrate their loved one's progress, further motivating them to continue making healthy choices.

It is important to note that family involvement and support should be balanced with respect for individual autonomy and personal choices. Each person's preferences and readiness for change may vary, so it's crucial to communicate and collaborate openly while being sensitive to their needs and boundaries.

Overall, family support plays an integral role in promoting and sustaining lifestyle changes for individuals with schizophrenia. By offering education, encouragement, creating a supportive environment, and actively participating in the journey, families can significantly enhance the individual's overall well-being and treatment outcomes.

Chapter 4: Caring for a Loved One with Schizophrenia

The Role of the Caregiver

Schizophrenia is a complex mental disorder that affects millions of people worldwide. The impact of schizophrenia extends beyond the individual diagnosed; it also affects their family and friends, particularly the primary caregiver.

The caregiver plays a pivotal role in supporting and promoting the well-being of their loved one with schizophrenia. This article aims to explore the challenges faced by caregivers and provide insights into their crucial responsibilities in caring for someone with schizophrenia.

Understanding Schizophrenia: Before delving into the caregiver's role, it is essential to develop a comprehensive understanding of schizophrenia. Schizophrenia is a chronic condition that requires ongoing management and treatment. The symptoms can be categorized into positive (delusions, hallucinations), negative (social withdrawal, decreased emotional expression), and cognitive (impaired thinking, memory problems) symptoms. Each individual's experience with schizophrenia is unique, making it important for caregivers to have a thorough understanding of the illness and its manifestations.

Emotional Impact on Caregivers: Caring for a loved one with schizophrenia can be emotionally challenging. Caregivers often experience a range of emotions such as stress, anxiety, guilt, and sadness. Witnessing their loved one's struggles, navigating the healthcare system, and dealing with the stigma associated with mental illness can take a toll on caregivers' mental health. It is crucial for caregivers to prioritize self-care and seek support from support groups or therapists to manage their emotions effectively.

Role of the Caregiver:

1. Education and Advocacy: One of the primary responsibilities of a caregiver is to educate themselves about schizophrenia. This knowledge equips them to understand the symptoms, treatment options, and available resources. By becoming informed advocates, caregivers can play an active role in their loved one's recovery journey.

2. Medication Management: Ensuring medication adherence is crucial in managing schizophrenia effectively. Caregivers play a vital role in helping their loved ones stick to their medication regimen. This can involve organizing pillboxes, setting reminders, and monitoring any side effects. They may also be required to accompany their loved one to medical appointments and communicate with healthcare professionals regularly.

3. Lifestyle Support: Promoting a healthy lifestyle is essential for individuals with schizophrenia. Caregivers can assist by encouraging regular exercise, a balanced diet, and adequate sleep. Creating a stable and structured routine can help manage symptoms and foster a sense of stability in their loved one's life. Additionally, caregivers can

provide emotional support, engaging in activities that promote socialization and reducing stress.

4. Crisis Management: Schizophrenia can sometimes involve episodes of crisis or relapse. Caregivers need to be prepared to manage these situations effectively. This may involve knowing the signs of relapse, having a crisis plan in place, and being in touch with emergency contacts and healthcare professionals. Caregivers should also be aware of resources available in the community, such as crisis hotlines and support services.

5. Communication and Social Interaction: Caregivers play a crucial role in facilitating social interaction for their loved ones with schizophrenia. Encouraging social connections, whether through family gatherings, support groups, or community activities, can help reduce feelings of isolation and improve overall well-being. Effective communication skills are essential in providing emotional support, active listening, and understanding their loved one's needs.

6. Coping Strategies and Emotional Support: Living with schizophrenia can be overwhelming for both the individual and their caregiver. Caregivers can help by teaching and practicing coping strategies for managing symptoms, stress, and anxiety. They can provide a safe and non-judgmental space for their loved ones to express their emotions and concerns. Caregivers should also be aware of available support groups and therapeutic

interventions that can provide additional emotional support.

7. Respite and Self-Care: Caring for a loved one with schizhrenia can be demanding, both physically and emotionally. It is vital for caregivers to prioritize self-care and seek respite when needed. Taking breaks, engaging in activities they enjoy, and seeking support from friends and family can prevent burnout and maintain their own well-being. Respite care options, such as temporary professional caregivers or support services, should be explored to ensure the caregiver receives the necessary rest and rejuvenation.

Conclusion: Caring for a loved one with schizophrenia is a challenging but essential role. The caregiver's responsibilities extend beyond mere physical care to encompass emotional support, advocacy, and crisis management. Understanding schizophrenia and its symptoms is key to providing effective care. While caregiving can be emotionally demanding, caregivers must prioritize self-care to maintain their own mental health. Support, education, and accessing available resources can help caregivers in their journey as they navigate the challenges and promote the well-being of their loved ones with schizophrenia.

Communication Strategies

Effective communication is crucial in any relationship, but it becomes even more essential when caring for a loved one with schizophrenia. Schizophrenia is a complex mental disorder that affects an individual's thinking, perception, and communication skills. Communication challenges can arise due to symptoms such as disorganized speech, difficulty concentrating, or impaired social interactions. This section aims to explore strategies for effective communication with a loved one with schizophrenia.

Understanding Communication Challenges in Schizophrenia:

To effectively communicate with a loved one with schizophrenia, it is essential to understand the common communication challenges they may face. These challenges can vary depending on the individual's symptoms and the severity of their condition. Some common communication challenges in schizophrenia include:

1. Disorganized Speech: Schizophrenia can cause disorganized thinking and speaking, making it difficult for individuals to express themselves clearly or make coherent statements. Their speech may appear illogical, tangential, or unrelated to the conversation at hand.

2. Hallucinations and Delusions: Individuals with schizophrenia may experience hallucinations (perceiving things that do not exist) or delusions (holding beliefs that are not based in reality). These experiences can make communication difficult as the individual may become preoccupied with their hallucinations or delusions, leading to misunderstandings or a lack of focus.

3. Social Withdrawal: Schizophrenia can cause individuals to withdraw from social interactions, leading to reduced communication or a lack of initiative in initiating conversations. They may prefer solitude or feel uncomfortable in social situations.

4. Cognitive Impairments: Schizophrenia can affect cognitive functions such as memory, attention, and problem-solving skills. This can make it challenging for individuals to process information, follow conversations, or understand complex ideas.

Communication Strategies:

1. Active Listening: Active listening involves fully focusing on and understanding what the individual is saying. It includes maintaining eye contact, nodding to show understanding, and avoiding distractions. Actively listening allows the caregiver to show empathy and validate their loved one's experiences.

2. Speak Clearly and Simply: When communicating with a loved one with schizophrenia, it is important to speak clearly and use simple language. Complex or abstract concepts may be challenging for them to understand. Breaking down information into smaller, more manageable parts can facilitate comprehension and reduce confusion.

3. Be Patient and Understanding: Patience is crucial when communicating with someone with schizophrenia. It is essential to allow extra time for

them to process information and formulate their responses. Avoid rushing or interrupting, as it can cause frustration or anxiety. Being understanding and empathetic can create a safe and supportive environment for communication.

4. Avoid Arguing or Challenging Delusions: When your loved one expresses delusional beliefs, it is essential to avoid arguing or directly challenging their perceptions. Engaging in arguments can escalate the situation and potentially worsen their symptoms. Instead, try to redirect the conversation to a neutral or positive topic and validate their emotions without endorsing their delusions.

5. Use Visual Aids or Written Instructions: Visual aids, such as charts, diagrams, or drawings, can assist in conveying information more effectively. Written instructions or lists can serve as reminders and help individuals with memory impairments. These strategies can enhance understanding and provide a visual reference for important information.

6. Break Tasks into Manageable Steps: Individuals with schizophrenia may struggle with initiating and completing tasks. Breaking tasks into smaller, manageable steps can help them navigate daily activities more successfully. Providing clear instructions and offering assistance can make tasks feel less overwhelming.

7. Use Non-Verbal Communication: Non-verbal communication, such as facial expressions,

gestures, and touch, can convey emotions and support empathy. Maintaining a calm and reassuring demeanor, using appropriate facial expressions, and providing gentle touch can help individuals feel understood and validated.

8. Maintain a Calm Environment: Creating a calm and quiet environment can minimize distractions and improve focus during conversations. Reducing external stimuli such as noise or bright lights can help individuals concentrate on the conversation and reduce anxiety or agitation.

9. Validate Emotions and Feelings: Individuals with schizophrenia may experience intense emotions. Validating their emotions and feelings can help establish trust and encourage open communication. Acknowledge their emotions, express empathy, and refrain from dismissing or minimizing their experiences.

10. Utilize Supportive Language: Choosing supportive language can enhance communication and foster a positive atmosphere. Use positive and encouraging words, avoid judgmental or critical language, and focus on strengths and accomplishments rather than shortcomings.

11. Seek Professional Guidance: In some cases, seeking professional assistance, such as family therapy or communication skills training, can be beneficial. Mental health professionals can provide guidance

specific to your loved one's needs and help navigate challenging communication situations.

Conclusion: Communication plays a vital role in caring for a loved one with schizophrenia. By understanding the communication challenges associated with schizophrenia, caregivers can employ effective strategies to foster meaningful connections and promote understanding. Active listening, clear and simple language, patience, and empathy are key elements in successful communication. By creating a supportive environment and utilizing appropriate techniques,

Creating a Supportive Environment

When caring for a loved one with schizophrenia, creating a supportive environment is crucial for their well-being and overall quality of life. Schizophrenia is a complex mental disorder characterized by a disruption in thinking, emotions, and perceptions. The symptoms can be challenging to manage, making it essential for caregivers to provide a safe, understanding, and supportive atmosphere. This article aims to explore strategies and principles for creating a supportive environment for individuals with schizophrenia.

Understanding Schizophrenia's Impact on the Environment: Schizophrenia can have a significant impact on an individual's functioning and relationships within the environment. The symptoms, such as hallucinations, delusions, disorganized thinking, and social withdrawal, can disrupt their ability to navigate and interact with their surroundings. This disruption can lead to increased stress, isolation, and difficulty in performing day-to-day activities.

By creating a supportive environment, caregivers can help reduce these challenges and enhance their loved one's sense of stability and well-being.

Principles for Creating a Supportive Environment:

1. Education and Awareness: Understanding and educating oneself about schizophrenia is the foundation for creating a supportive environment. Learning about the disorder, its symptoms, and treatment options can help caregivers develop empathy, reduce stigma, and provide informed support. Education can also help family members and friends understand the challenges their loved one faces and provide appropriate assistance.

2. Empathy and Non-Judgment: A supportive environment must be built on empathy and non-judgmental attitudes. Caregivers should strive to understand their loved one's experiences, emotions, and perceptions, even if they may seem illogical or disconnected from reality. By withholding judgment and focusing on empathy, caregivers can establish a foundation of trust and open communication.

3. Clear Communication: Effective communication is essential for maintaining a supportive environment. Caregivers should strive to communicate clearly and directly, using simple and concise language. Avoiding ambiguous or confusing messages can promote understanding and reduce

stress. Nonverbal communication, such as facial expressions and gestures, can also enhance comprehension and emotional connection.

4. Structure and Routine: Individuals with schizophrenia often benefit from structured routines. Establishing regular daily activities, including sleeping, eating, and engaging in meaningful occupations, can provide a sense of predictability and stability. Caregivers should work together with their loved ones to create a schedule that suits their needs and abilities, taking into account their preferences and limitations.

5. Physical Safety: Ensuring physical safety is crucial in caring for a loved one with schizophrenia. Caregivers should identify and address any potential hazards or risks in the environment. This may involve securing medications, removing objects that could be used to harm oneself or others, and implementing safety measures such as locks or alarms as needed. Regular assessments of the environment's safety can provide peace of mind for both the caregiver and the individual with schizophrenia.

6. Emotional Support: Building emotional support within the environment is vital for individuals with schizophrenia. Caregivers should create a space where their loved ones feel comfortable expressing their emotions, concerns, and fears. Offering reassurance, active listening, and validation can help alleviate distress and promote emotional well-

being. Encouraging the person to engage in activities they enjoy can also foster positivity and a sense of accomplishment.

7. Social Interaction: Maintaining social connections is crucial for individuals with schizophrenia, as social withdrawal is often a symptom of the disorder. Caregivers should actively support their loved ones in engaging with their social networks, whether it be through family activities, support groups, or community events. Providing opportunities for social interaction can reduce feelings of loneliness and isolation, enhance self-esteem, and promote a sense of belonging.

8. Access to Treatment and Support Services: Creating a supportive environment involves facilitating access to necessary treatments and support services. Caregivers should work closely with healthcare professionals to ensure that their loved ones receive appropriate medications, therapies, and interventions. This may involve accompanying them to medical appointments, advocating for their needs, and staying informed about available community resources and support groups.

9. Encouraging Independence and Autonomy: While support is essential, caregivers should also foster independence and autonomy. Encouraging their loved ones to participate in decision-making, problem-solving, and activities of daily living can promote a sense of self-efficacy and empowerment. Caregivers should aim to strike a

balance between providing support and allowing their loved ones to take ownership of their lives.

10. Self-Care for Caregivers: Creating a supportive environment involves caring for the caregiver as well. Caregivers should prioritize their own self-care to maintain their own well-being. This may involve seeking support from other family members, friends, or support groups. Taking breaks, engaging in activities they enjoy, and acknowledging their own emotional needs are essential for preventing burnout and maintaining a supportive environment for their loved one.

Creating a supportive environment is crucial when caring for a loved one with schizophrenia. By developing an understanding of the disorder, adopting empathetic attitudes, and implementing effective strategies, caregivers can help promote a sense of stability, safety, and well-being for their loved one. Clear communication, structured routines, and emotional support are key elements in creating a supportive environment. It is also important to facilitate social interactions, ensure access to treatment and support services, and encourage independence and autonomy. Lastly, caregivers should prioritize their own self-care to maintain their own well-being as they navigate the challenges of caring for a loved one with schizophrenia. By implementing these principles, caregivers can positively impact their loved one's daily life and contribute to their overall recovery and quality of life.

Chapter 5: Navigating the Healthcare System

Seeking Help: Where to Start?

Navigating the healthcare system can be a daunting task, especially when trying to find help for a loved one suspected of having schizophrenia. Knowing where to start is crucial for getting the support and treatment needed. This section provides guidance on the initial steps to take, ensuring a pathway towards effective care.

Recognizing the Need for Professional Help

The first step in seeking help is recognizing the signs and symptoms that might indicate the presence of schizophrenia or another psychiatric condition. Early signs can include withdrawal from social situations, unusual behavior, expressions of strange thoughts or delusions, and hearing or seeing things that others do not. Acknowledging these signs and understanding the need for professional evaluation is critical.

Primary Care Physician (PCP)

A primary care physician (PCP) can be a good starting point. They can assess the individual's overall health, rule out other conditions that might mimic psychiatric disorders, and provide referrals to mental health specialists. Be open and thorough in describing the symptoms and behaviors observed, as this will assist the PCP in making an informed decision regarding the next steps.

Mental Health Professionals

Mental health professionals, including psychiatrists, psychologists, and psychiatric nurses, specialize in diagnosing and treating mental health conditions. A psychiatrist, in particular, can evaluate symptoms, make a diagnosis, and prescribe medication if necessary. Psychologists and therapists can offer psychotherapy to help manage symptoms and improve quality of life.

- **Psychiatrists**: Medical doctors who specialize in mental health and are qualified to prescribe medication.

- **Psychologists**: Professionals who specialize in psychotherapy but cannot prescribe medication in most jurisdictions.

- **Licensed Clinical Social Workers (LCSWs) and Licensed Professional Counselors (LPCs)**: Provide therapy and support for individuals and families.

Referral Networks and Support Organizations

Many organizations and networks can help connect you with mental health professionals and services. National and local mental health associations often maintain directories of mental health providers and offer resources for families and individuals facing mental health challenges. Examples include the National Alliance on Mental Illness (NAMI) in the United States and similar organizations worldwide.

Community Mental Health Centers

Community mental health centers provide access to mental health services, including assessment, treatment, and support services, often at a reduced cost or on a sliding scale based on income. These centers can be vital resources for individuals without insurance or with limited financial resources.

Crisis Services

In situations where there is a risk of harm to oneself or others, it's important to know how to access emergency services:

- **Emergency Rooms**: For immediate crises, the emergency room can provide urgent assessment and safety.

- **Crisis Hotlines**: National and local hotlines offer support and guidance on immediate steps to take in a crisis.

Insurance Considerations

Understanding your insurance coverage is essential for accessing services. Contact your insurance provider to inquire about covered services, including psychiatric evaluations, therapy sessions, and medication. Insurance plans vary widely, so knowing the specifics can help in planning treatment.

Navigating the healthcare system requires persistence, advocacy, and informed decision-making. Starting with a primary care physician, leveraging mental health professionals, utilizing support networks, and understanding insurance coverage are key steps in securing the necessary support and treatment for schizophrenia. This process underscores the importance of advocating for your loved one's health and well-being within the healthcare system.

Long-Term Planning

After taking the initial steps to enter the healthcare system and securing initial assessments and treatments, families and caregivers must engage in advanced navigation and long-term planning to ensure ongoing support for their loved ones with schizophrenia. This phase involves deeper engagement with mental health services, leveraging specialized programs, and planning for long-term care and support.

Engaging with Specialized Mental Health Services

As treatment progresses, it may become necessary to engage with more specialized mental health services, including those offered by psychiatrists who specialize in schizophrenia, early psychosis intervention programs, and specialized outpatient services. These services often provide comprehensive care tailored to the specific needs of individuals with schizophrenia, including medication management, psychotherapy, family therapy, and support for education and employment.

Early Psychosis Intervention Programs

Early intervention in psychosis, particularly during the first episode, can significantly impact long-term outcomes. These programs specialize in treating individuals in the early stages of psychosis, offering a range of medical, psychological, and social interventions designed to reduce symptoms, prevent relapse, and support recovery. If your loved one is in the early stages of schizophrenia, seeking out these programs can be particularly beneficial.

Specialized Outpatient Services

For ongoing treatment, specialized outpatient services can offer consistent support tailored to the needs of those with schizophrenia. These may include assertive community treatment (ACT) teams, day programs, and vocational rehabilitation services. These services aim to maintain stability, prevent hospitalization, and support individuals in living as independently as possible.

Planning for Long-Term Care and Support

Long-term care planning is essential for ensuring that individuals with schizophrenia have the support they need over time. This planning may involve:

- **Legal and Financial Planning**: Establishing power of attorney, setting up special needs trusts, and planning for financial security are important steps to protect your loved one's future.

- **Housing Options**: Exploring safe and supportive living arrangements, such as supported housing programs or group homes, can provide stable environments conducive to managing schizophrenia.

- **Continuity of Care**: Ensuring ongoing access to mental health services and medical care is crucial for long-term management. This may involve coordinating care among different providers and services and advocating for comprehensive care coverage.

- **Support Networks**: Building and maintaining a network of support, including family, friends, peer support groups, and mental health organizations, can provide invaluable resources and emotional support for both individuals with schizophrenia and their families.

Working with Healthcare Professionals

Effective collaboration with healthcare professionals is crucial in managing schizophrenia. Building a strong, cooperative relationship with your loved one's care team can significantly impact their treatment journey, ensuring they receive comprehensive and personalized care. Here are key strategies for working effectively with healthcare professionals:

Building a Relationship Based on Trust and Respect

- **Open Communication**: Establish open lines of communication with healthcare providers. Be honest and thorough in sharing observations, concerns, and questions regarding your loved one's condition and treatment. Encourage your loved one to communicate openly with their care team, too.

- **Respect Expertise**: While it's important to be an advocate for your loved one, also respect the expertise and experience of healthcare professionals. Balancing advocacy with respect helps foster a productive partnership.

Participating Actively in Treatment Decisions

- **Informed Decision-Making**: Educate yourself about schizophrenia, including treatment options and potential side effects of medications. This knowledge will empower you to participate actively in treatment decisions.

- **Collaborative Care Planning**: Work with healthcare providers to develop a care plan that addresses both the medical and personal needs of your loved one. Ensure the plan is realistic and consider your loved one's preferences and lifestyle.

Advocating for Your Loved One's Needs

- **Advocacy**: Be prepared to advocate for your loved one's needs, ensuring they receive the best possible care. This may involve asking for second opinions, inquiring about alternative treatments, or seeking additional support services.

- **Insurance Navigation**: Understand your insurance coverage and be prepared to navigate its complexities. This may involve discussing treatment plans with insurance representatives or appealing denied coverage for certain treatments.

Ensuring Continuity of Care

- **Care Coordination**: Schizophrenia treatment often involves multiple professionals, including psychiatrists, psychologists, social workers, and possibly other specialists. Strive to ensure that all members of the care team are informed about treatment plans and progress, facilitating coordinated care.

- **Record Keeping**: Keep detailed records of treatments, medications, hospitalizations, and interactions with healthcare providers. This information can be invaluable in managing your loved one's care, particularly when transitioning between providers or evaluating treatment effectiveness.

Addressing Setbacks and Challenges

- **Flexibility**: Be prepared for setbacks and changes in the treatment plan. Schizophrenia can be unpredictable, and adjustments to the treatment approach may be necessary.

- **Support Networks**: Utilize support networks, including support groups for families of individuals with schizophrenia. These groups can provide practical advice, emotional support, and insights from others who have navigated similar challenges.

Encouraging Independence and Self-Advocacy

- **Empowerment**: Encourage your loved one to take an active role in their treatment when possible. This promotes independence and self-advocacy, important components of recovery and self-management.

- **Education**: Support your loved one in learning about their condition and treatment options. Knowledge can empower them to make informed decisions about their care and advocate for their own needs.

Working with healthcare professionals in a collaborative, respectful manner is essential for the effective management of schizophrenia. By actively participating in the care process, advocating for your loved one, and fostering open communication, families can help ensure that their loved ones receive the comprehensive and personalized care necessary for their well-being and recovery.

Advocacy and Legal Rights

Advocacy for individuals with schizophrenia involves both personal advocacy for oneself or a loved one and broader advocacy for the rights and dignity of all individuals with mental health conditions. Understanding and asserting legal rights is a critical component of this advocacy. It ensures access to necessary treatments, services, and supports while protecting individuals from discrimination and stigma. Here's how to approach advocacy and understand legal rights:

Personal Advocacy

- **Educate Yourself**: Knowledge about schizophrenia, treatment options, and the mental health system empowers you to make informed decisions and advocate effectively.

- **Build a Support Network**: Connecting with others through support groups and mental health organizations can provide valuable insights, resources, and collective advocacy opportunities.

- **Communicate Effectively**: Develop clear communication with healthcare providers, expressing needs, preferences, and concerns while also listening to professional advice and options.

- **Document Everything**: Keep detailed records of treatments, communications with healthcare providers, and any legal documents related to care. This information can be crucial for advocacy and legal matters.

Legal Rights

Understanding and navigating legal rights is vital for protecting and advocating for individuals with schizophrenia.

Right to Treatment

- **Access to Care**: Individuals have the right to accessible, appropriate, and humane treatment for mental health conditions, including schizophrenia. This includes the right to be informed about treatment options and to participate in treatment decisions.

- **Confidentiality**: Patients have a right to privacy regarding their medical condition and treatment. Information cannot be disclosed without consent, except in specific legal or emergency situations.

Right to Refuse Treatment

- **Informed Consent**: Patients have the right to informed consent, meaning they must be informed about the benefits and risks of treatment and alternatives. They also have the right to refuse treatment, except in cases where they pose a significant risk to themselves or others.

Rights in the Workplace

- **Anti-Discrimination Laws**: Laws such as the Americans with Disabilities Act (ADA) in the U.S. protect individuals with disabilities, including mental health conditions, from discrimination in employment. Employers are required to provide reasonable accommodations to qualified individuals.

- **Family Medical Leave Act (FMLA)**: In the U.S., this act allows eligible employees to take unpaid, job-protected leave for specified family and medical reasons, including caring for a family member with a serious health condition.

Housing Rights

- **Fair Housing Act**: This act protects people from discrimination when renting or buying a home, getting a mortgage, seeking housing assistance, or engaging in other housing-related activities. It includes protections for individuals with disabilities, including those with mental health conditions.

Systemic Advocacy

- **Policy Change**: Engaging in advocacy at the policy level can help bring about changes that improve access to care, funding for mental health services, and protections for individuals with mental health conditions.

- **Public Awareness**: Raising public awareness about schizophrenia and mental health can help reduce stigma and misinformation, creating a more informed and compassionate society.

Advocacy and understanding legal rights are crucial for navigating the complexities of living with schizophrenia, ensuring that individuals and their families have access to necessary support and are treated with dignity and respect.

it's important to explore additional facets of advocating for individuals with schizophrenia, focusing on education, community involvement, and navigating the criminal justice system. These areas underscore the comprehensive approach needed to support individuals with mental health conditions effectively.

Educational Rights

Individuals with schizophrenia, especially younger patients who are in educational settings, have rights that need to be respected and upheld:

- **Individuals with Disabilities Education Act (IDEA)**: In the United States, this act requires public schools to provide free appropriate public education (FAPE) in the least restrictive environment to children with disabilities, including those with serious mental health conditions.

- **Section 504 of the Rehabilitation Act**: This civil rights law prohibits discrimination against individuals with disabilities in programs that receive federal financial assistance, including public schools, universities, and other educational institutions. It ensures that students with disabilities have equal access to education and may include accommodations tailored to their needs.

Community Involvement and Social Inclusion

Advocacy extends beyond the individual and legal realms into community involvement and social inclusion:

- **Participation in Community Life**: Advocacy efforts can focus on ensuring that individuals with schizophrenia have opportunities to participate fully in community life, including access to recreational activities, volunteer opportunities, and social events.

- **Social Inclusion Initiatives**: Programs aimed at integrating individuals with mental health conditions into community activities can help reduce isolation and stigma. Advocates can support policies and programs that promote inclusion and understanding within communities.

Navigating the Criminal Justice System

Individuals with schizophrenia occasionally come into contact with the criminal justice system, making advocacy in this area crucial:

- **Mental Health Courts**: These specialized court docket programs are designed for individuals with mental health conditions who are involved in the criminal justice system. They aim to offer treatment and support instead of traditional incarceration, focusing on rehabilitation.

- **Legal Representation**: Ensuring that individuals with schizophrenia have access to legal representation knowledgeable about mental health issues is critical, especially in cases where their condition may impact their legal situation.

- **Training for Law Enforcement**: Advocating for training programs for law enforcement personnel on how to recognize and appropriately respond to individuals with mental health conditions can help prevent misunderstandings and ensure safer interactions.

Long-Term Care and Guardianship

In some cases, individuals with schizophrenia may require long-term care planning or guardianship arrangements:

- **Advance Directives for Mental Health**: These are legal documents that allow individuals to outline their preferences for treatment in case they are unable to make decisions for themselves in the future. Advocating for the use of advance directives can ensure that a person's treatment preferences are respected.

- **Guardianship**: In situations where an individual is unable to make decisions for themselves, families may consider guardianship. It's important to understand the legal implications and responsibilities involved in becoming a guardian, as well as alternative options that might offer more autonomy to the individual.

Advocacy for individuals with schizophrenia is a multifaceted effort that encompasses personal, legal, educational, and community domains. By understanding and utilizing the tools and resources available, advocates can work towards ensuring that individuals with schizophrenia receive the respect, care, and support they need to lead fulfilling lives. This advocacy not only benefits individuals with schizophrenia but also contributes to a more inclusive, compassionate, and informed society.

Chapter 6: Self-Care for Caregivers

Coping Mechanisms

Focusing specifically on coping mechanisms for caregivers, it's vital to recognize that caregiving, while deeply rewarding, can also be a source of significant stress. Effective coping mechanisms can help caregivers manage stress, avoid burnout, and maintain their well-being. Here are some targeted strategies for caregivers to cope with the demands of caring for a loved one with schizophrenia:

Develop a Self-Care Routine

- **Routine Physical Activity**: Engage in regular exercise, which is proven to reduce stress, improve mood, and boost physical health. Even short, daily walks can make a significant difference.

- **Balanced Diet**: Eating a healthy, balanced diet supports physical health and can affect your mood and energy levels.

- **Adequate Sleep**: Prioritize getting enough sleep, as sleep deprivation can exacerbate stress and negatively impact health.

Practice Mindfulness and Relaxation Techniques

- **Mindfulness Meditation**: Practicing mindfulness can help you stay grounded in the present moment, reducing stress and anxiety.

- **Deep Breathing Exercises**: Simple breathing techniques can calm the nervous system and provide a quick way to reduce stress in moments of high tension.

- **Progressive Muscle Relaxation (PMR)**: This technique involves tensing and then relaxing different muscle groups in the body, promoting physical and mental relaxation.

Set Boundaries and Manage Time

- **Learn to Say No**: It's crucial to recognize your limits and avoid overcommitting. Saying no is a necessary part of self-care.

- **Time Management**: Use time management strategies to balance caregiving duties with personal time. This can include setting aside specific times for relaxation and activities you enjoy.

Seek and Accept Support

- **Support Networks**: Connect with support groups or online forums for caregivers. Sharing experiences with others in similar situations can provide emotional support and practical advice.

- **Accept Help**: Don't hesitate to accept offers of help from friends, family, or community services. Delegating tasks can provide you with much-needed breaks.

Engage in Activities That Bring Joy

- **Hobbies and Interests**: Continue to engage in hobbies and activities that bring you pleasure.

These activities can provide a welcome escape and help maintain your identity beyond your role as a caregiver.

Keep a Journal

- **Reflective Writing**: Keeping a journal can be a therapeutic way to express feelings, reflect on experiences, and celebrate successes. Writing about your caregiving journey can help process emotions and reduce stress.

Professional Support

- **Counseling or Therapy**: Consider seeking professional support if you find yourself overwhelmed. Therapists can offer coping strategies and provide a safe space to discuss your feelings and challenges.

Educate Yourself

- **Learn About Schizophrenia**: Understanding the condition can demystify your loved one's behaviors and help you respond more effectively. Knowledge can empower you and reduce feelings of helplessness.

Maintain Perspective

- **Focus on What You Can Control**: Recognize that some aspects of schizophrenia and caregiving are beyond your control. Focusing on what you can influence can help reduce feelings of frustration.

Practice Gratitude

- **Gratitude Journaling**: Regularly noting things you're grateful for can shift focus from the challenges of caregiving to the positive aspects of your life, enhancing overall well-being.

Adopting these coping mechanisms can help caregivers maintain their health and well-being, ensuring they are better equipped to care for their loved ones with schizophrenia. Remember, taking care of yourself is not an act of selfishness; it's a necessity for providing compassionate and effective care.

Balancing Caregiving with Personal Life

Balancing caregiving responsibilities with personal life is crucial for maintaining the well-being of caregivers. The intense demands of caring for a loved one with schizophrenia can sometimes overshadow personal needs, leading to burnout and diminished quality of life. Here are strategies to help caregivers find a balance between these important aspects of their lives:

Prioritize Self-Care

Self-care is Non-negotiable: Recognize that taking care of your health and well-being is not optional—it's essential. This includes physical health through exercise and nutrition, mental health through stress management and hobbies, and emotional health through social connections and downtime.

Establish a Routine

Create a Structured Schedule: Develop a daily and weekly routine that includes time allocated for caregiving tasks, personal activities, work, and rest. A structured schedule can help manage stress and prevent caregiver burnout by ensuring personal time is not neglected.

Set Boundaries

Define Limits: Clearly define what you are willing and able to do in your caregiving role, and communicate these boundaries to others. Setting boundaries helps manage expectations and prevents resentment and exhaustion.

Delegate and Share Responsibilities

Seek Help: You don't have to do everything yourself. Identify tasks that can be delegated to other family members, friends, or professional caregivers. Sharing the load can free up time for your personal needs and interests.

Utilize Respite Care Services

Take Breaks: Respite care provides temporary relief for caregivers, offering services such as in-home care or short-term facility care for your loved one. Utilizing respite care allows you to take breaks, recharge, and tend to personal matters without worry.

Maintain Social Connections

Stay Connected: Keep in touch with friends and participate in social activities. Social support is vital for emotional well-being and can provide an important outlet outside of caregiving responsibilities.

Pursue Personal Interests and Hobbies

Keep Your Identity: It's important to maintain your own identity beyond being a caregiver. Continue to engage in hobbies, interests, and personal goals that bring you joy and fulfillment.

Communicate Needs

Open Communication: Clearly communicate your needs and feelings to family members and friends. Letting others know when you need support can help balance caregiving and personal life.

Practice Mindful Acceptance

Accept What You Cannot Change: Some aspects of caregiving and schizophrenia cannot be changed. Practicing acceptance can help reduce stress and promote a focus on the present moment, enhancing your ability to enjoy personal time.

Plan for the Future

Long-term Planning: Engage in long-term planning for your loved one's care. Knowing there's a plan in place can reduce anxiety about the future, allowing you to enjoy the present more fully.

Seek Professional Guidance

Counseling: If balancing caregiving and personal life becomes overwhelming, consider seeking professional advice from a counselor or therapist. They can offer strategies for coping and maintaining balance.

Celebrate Achievements

Acknowledge Your Efforts: Recognize and celebrate the hard work you do as a caregiver. Acknowledging your achievements can boost morale and remind you of the importance of balancing this role with your personal life.

Balancing caregiving with personal life requires intentionality, support, and self-compassion. By implementing these strategies, caregivers can ensure they maintain their own well-being while providing compassionate care for their loved ones with schizophrenia. This balance is crucial for sustaining the caregiving journey over the long term.

Seeking Support and Respite

Seeking support and respite is a critical aspect of self-care for caregivers. Caring for a loved one with schizophrenia is a marathon, not a sprint, and requires a sustainable approach that includes periods of rest and rejuvenation. Here's how caregivers can seek the support and respite they need to maintain their well-being and continue providing care effectively.

Understand the Importance of Respite

Acknowledge the Need for Breaks: Recognize that taking breaks is not a sign of weakness or lack of commitment. Instead, it's an essential component of a sustainable caregiving strategy that benefits both the caregiver and the person receiving care.

Explore Respite Care Options

Informal Support: Reach out to friends, family, or community members who can provide temporary care or assistance. Sometimes, informal support networks can offer significant relief.

Professional Respite Services: Investigate professional respite services available in your area. These can range from in-home care providers who offer short-term relief to specialized respite programs that allow for longer breaks.

Adult Day Care Centers: For individuals with schizophrenia who have some level of independence, adult day care centers can provide a safe environment for socialization and activities, offering caregivers a regular, predictable break.

Leverage Support Groups

Join Caregiver Support Groups: Support groups for caregivers of individuals with mental illness can provide emotional support, practical advice, and a sense of community. Sharing experiences with others who understand can be incredibly validating and helpful.

Online Forums and Communities: If in-person groups are not accessible, online forums and communities can also offer support and connection. These platforms allow you to seek advice and support at any time, from anywhere.

Utilize Community Resources

Mental Health Organizations: Organizations such as the National Alliance on Mental Illness (NAMI) offer resources, support, and educational programs for caregivers. These organizations can also help connect you with local respite care options.

Government and Nonprofit Programs: Research government and nonprofit programs that offer support services for caregivers, including respite care, counseling, and financial assistance.

Prioritize Emotional Support

Seek Professional Help: If the emotional burden of caregiving becomes overwhelming, consider seeking help from a mental health professional. Therapists or counselors can provide coping strategies and support to navigate the challenges of caregiving.

Maintain Personal Relationships: Keep up with personal relationships outside of your caregiving duties. Friends and family can provide emotional support and a much-needed break from caregiving responsibilities.

Educate Yourself

Stay Informed: Knowledge is empowering. Educating yourself about schizophrenia and caregiving strategies can help you feel more in control and less isolated. Many organizations offer workshops, seminars, and literature on caregiving.

Make Use of Technology

Utilize Apps and Online Tools: There are numerous apps and online tools designed to support caregivers, from organizing care schedules to managing medication reminders. These tools can help streamline caregiving tasks, freeing up time for rest and self-care.

Schedule Regular Breaks

Plan Ahead: Proactively schedule regular breaks and respite care into your routine. Knowing you have scheduled time off can help reduce stress and give you something to look forward to.

Communicate Your Needs

Open Dialogue: Communicate your need for support and respite with other family members and involved healthcare professionals. Being clear about your limits and needs can help ensure you receive the support you require.

Seeking support and respite is not a luxury—it's a necessity for caregivers. By taking steps to ensure you have regular breaks and a supportive network, you can protect your health and well-being, ultimately providing better care for your loved one with schizophrenia.

Chapter 7: Living with Schizophrenia 2

Stories of Recognition, Diagnosis, Treatment, and Family Support

This chapter unfolds the deeply personal and often profound journey of individuals with schizophrenia and their families, from the initial recognition of symptoms through to diagnosis, the challenges and successes of treatment, and the crucial role of family support. Each narrative is structured to reflect the logical sequence of these stages, providing insight into the lived experience of schizophrenia and highlighting the resilience and hope that emerge from adversity.

Story 1: Emma's Journey to Understanding

Recognition: Emma was in her late teens when her family first noticed signs that something was amiss. She began withdrawing from friends and family, expressing unusual thoughts, and appearing fearful of things that others couldn't see or hear.

Diagnosis: After several months of confusion and concern, Emma's parents encouraged her to see a psychiatrist. The process was fraught with anxiety, but eventually, she was diagnosed with schizophrenia. The diagnosis was a shock to Emma and her family but also brought a sense of relief in finally having a name for what was happening.

Treatment: Emma's treatment began with a combination of antipsychotic medication and cognitive behavioral therapy. The road was bumpy, with several medication adjustments needed to find the right balance for her.

Throughout this process, her family was her constant support system, helping her adhere to her treatment plan and encouraging her to stay engaged with her therapy sessions.

Family Support: Emma's family played a pivotal role in her journey. They educated themselves about schizophrenia, joined a support group for families, and learned how to communicate effectively with Emma about her experiences. Their unwavering support and love were crucial in helping Emma navigate the challenges of schizophrenia.

Story 2: David's Path to Recovery

Recognition: In his early twenties, David started experiencing profound changes in his behavior and perception. He heard voices that no one else could hear and held beliefs that made little sense to those around him.

Diagnosis: After a particularly frightening episode of psychosis, David was admitted to a psychiatric hospital, where he was diagnosed with schizophrenia. The diagnosis was a critical turning point for him and his family, marking the start of his journey toward recovery.

Treatment: David's treatment initially focused on managing his psychotic symptoms through medication, which was later supplemented with psychotherapy to address the social and emotional aspects of his condition. Through trial and error, David and his healthcare team found a treatment regimen that worked for him.

Family Support: David's family was instrumental in his recovery. They worked closely with his healthcare providers to understand his needs and ensure he had the support necessary at home. They also became advocates for mental health awareness, sharing their story to help destigmatize schizophrenia.

Story 3: Sarah and the Power of Early Intervention

Recognition: Sarah's family knew little about schizophrenia until her behavior dramatically changed during her first year of college, marked by paranoia and disorganized thinking.

Diagnosis: With the encouragement of her family, Sarah sought help early, leading to a prompt diagnosis. The early recognition of her symptoms was crucial in accessing treatment before her condition worsened.

Treatment: Sarah benefited from an early intervention program specializing in first-episode psychosis, which offered a comprehensive approach to care, including medication management, psychoeducation, and family therapy. This early and aggressive approach to treatment was key to her successful management of schizophrenia.

Family Support: Sarah's family was closely involved in her treatment from the start. They participated in family therapy sessions, which helped improve their understanding of schizophrenia and how to support Sarah. Their commitment to her well-being was a constant source of strength for her.

Story 4: Michael's Road to Self-Acceptance

Recognition: Michael started showing signs of schizophrenia in his mid-twenties, characterized by severe social withdrawal and delusional thinking that alienated him from his peers. His performance at work suffered, and he became increasingly isolated.

Diagnosis: It took a crisis situation for Michael's family to intervene and seek psychiatric help for him. After an acute psychotic episode, he was hospitalized and diagnosed with schizophrenia. The diagnosis was a difficult pill to swallow for Michael, who had little understanding of mental health conditions.

Treatment: Michael's treatment plan included antipsychotic medications to manage his symptoms and cognitive-behavioral therapy (CBT) to help him deal with the underlying thought patterns contributing to his condition. It was a gradual process, but over time, Michael began to see improvements in his thought processes and social interactions.

Family Support: Initially resistant to his family's efforts to help, Michael eventually came to appreciate their persistence and dedication. They became his biggest advocates, supporting him through the ups and downs of his treatment. Their involvement in his care plan and their efforts to educate themselves about schizophrenia were crucial in helping Michael come to terms with his condition and work towards recovery.

Story 5: Linda's Lifelong Journey with Schizophrenia

Recognition: Linda was diagnosed with schizophrenia in her late teens, following years of battling with hallucinations and disorganized thoughts that made her high school years incredibly challenging.

Diagnosis: After multiple visits to different healthcare providers, Linda was finally diagnosed with schizophrenia. The diagnosis came as a relief to Linda and her family, as it provided a name to her experiences and a path forward for treatment.

Treatment: Over the decades, Linda has been on various treatment regimens, experiencing the evolution of schizophrenia treatment firsthand—from the early use of first-generation antipsychotics to the more recent and tolerable second-generation medications. Alongside pharmacotherapy, Linda has consistently participated in psychotherapy, which has been instrumental in helping her manage her symptoms and maintain her independence.

Family Support: Linda's family has been her cornerstone, providing unwavering support throughout her life. They've navigated the changing landscape of mental health care together, advocating for Linda's rights and ensuring she has access to the best available treatments. Their commitment has been a constant source of hope and stability for Linda, allowing her to lead a fulfilling life despite the challenges of schizophrenia.

Story 6: The Williams Family: Navigating Schizophrenia Together

Recognition: When the Williams' youngest son, Tom, began exhibiting erratic behavior and expressing bizarre and paranoid thoughts, they knew something was seriously wrong. His transition from adolescence to adulthood was marked by increasing signs of psychosis.

Diagnosis: After a series of assessments, Tom was diagnosed with schizophrenia. The diagnosis was a pivotal moment for the family, forcing them to confront the reality of mental illness and its implications.

Treatment: The family embarked on a comprehensive treatment plan for Tom, including medication management, individual therapy, and family counseling. They learned the importance of a coordinated approach to care, addressing not just the symptoms but the social and emotional aspects of Tom's life.

Family Support: The Williams family's journey was characterized by their collective effort to support Tom. They educated themselves about schizophrenia, connected with support groups, and worked tirelessly to provide a nurturing and understanding environment for Tom. Their story highlights the power of family unity and the positive impact it can have on the individual's coping and recovery process.

These personal narratives further enrich our understanding of the schizophrenia journey, emphasizing the diverse experiences of individuals and their families. From the struggles of coming to terms with the diagnosis to the triumphs of finding effective treatment and support, each story offers unique insights into the resilience and strength required to navigate this condition. The common thread through all these stories is the indispensable role of understanding, acceptance, and support—whether from family, friends, or the wider community—in fostering hope and facilitating recovery.

Key takeaways from the Personal Narratives

Drawing from the personal narratives shared in the previous discussions, we can identify key lessons learned and advice from each story, offering a deeper dive into the insights gained from their experiences with schizophrenia.

Emma's Journey to Understanding

Key Takeaway: The importance of family support and early intervention in the treatment process. Emma's story highlights how recognizing the signs of schizophrenia early and seeking professional help promptly can lead to a more manageable treatment journey.

Advice: Encourage families to act quickly when symptoms arise and to approach the situation with empathy and understanding. Building a strong support system around the individual can significantly impact their ability to cope with and manage their condition.

David's Path to Recovery

Key Takeaway: The value of persistence in finding the right treatment regimen. David's narrative illustrates that while the path to effective treatment can be fraught with challenges, perseverance pays off. Adjusting medications and therapy approaches is a common part of the process.

Advice: Remain patient and open to changes in the treatment plan. Effective management of schizophrenia often requires adjustments and can take time to achieve optimal results. Communication with healthcare providers is crucial in this iterative process.

Sarah and the Power of Early Intervention

Key Takeaway: The transformative impact of early intervention programs for schizophrenia. Sarah's experience underscores how accessing specialized treatment early, especially during the first episode of psychosis, can significantly improve long-term outcomes.

Advice: For individuals showing early signs of psychosis, seek out early intervention programs that offer comprehensive care, including medication management, psychoeducation, and support for both the individual and their family.

Michael's Road to Self-Acceptance

Key Takeaway: The journey towards self-acceptance and the critical role of personalized treatment plans. Michael's story reveals how understanding and accepting one's condition is a pivotal step in the recovery process, facilitated by a treatment plan tailored to the individual's specific needs.

Advice: Support loved ones in their journey toward accepting their diagnosis. Work collaboratively with healthcare providers to tailor treatment plans that respect the individual's goals, preferences, and lifestyle.

Linda's Lifelong Journey with Schizophrenia

Key Takeaway: The evolving nature of schizophrenia treatment and the necessity of continuous care. Linda's decades-long experience with schizophrenia demonstrates the importance of adapting to changes in treatment practices and the need for ongoing management of the condition.

Advice: Stay informed about the latest developments in schizophrenia treatment and be prepared to adjust care plans as new options become available. Long-term management of schizophrenia requires flexibility and an open dialogue between the individual, their family, and their care team.

The Williams Family: Navigating Schizophrenia Together

Key Takeaway: The strength of family unity in facing the challenges of schizophrenia. The Williams family's story emphasizes how a united front can significantly ease the burden of navigating schizophrenia, from diagnosis through treatment.

Advice: Foster strong family involvement in the care process. Educate the entire family about schizophrenia, and engage in joint therapy sessions when possible to improve communication, understanding, and support within the family unit.

Conclusion

These personal narratives and the lessons drawn from them illuminate the multifaceted challenges and triumphs faced by individuals with schizophrenia and their families. The overarching advice emphasizes early intervention, persistence in finding the right treatment, the power of family support, the necessity of self-care, and the importance of adapting to ongoing changes in the condition and its management. Each story serves as a beacon of hope and a guide for others on similar paths, showcasing that while schizophrenia is a complex and challenging condition, with the right support and strategies, individuals can lead fulfilling lives.

Maintaining Optimism and Forward Momentum

In the journey with schizophrenia, fostering hope is not just a passive state of wishing for the best; it's an active pursuit of optimism and forward momentum. This chapter explores strategies for maintaining hope and positive outlooks, both for individuals with schizophrenia and their families, underscoring the belief that despite the challenges, progress and recovery are possible.

Cultivating a Positive Outlook

Embrace Small Victories: Celebrate every step forward, no matter how small. Recognizing and valuing progress helps maintain momentum and builds confidence in the possibility of further improvements.

Set Realistic Goals: Setting achievable, incremental goals can provide a sense of purpose and direction. These goals can be related to treatment adherence, daily activities, or personal ambitions.

Leveraging Support Networks

Connect with Others: Joining support groups or communities of individuals and families navigating schizophrenia can be incredibly uplifting. These connections provide a platform to share experiences, strategies, and words of encouragement.

Engage in Peer Support: For individuals with schizophrenia, engaging with peer support workers who have lived experience of mental health conditions can be particularly empowering. They offer a unique perspective and understanding, fostering a sense of hope and possibility.

Focusing on Wellness

Holistic Health Approaches: Encourage practices that promote overall well-being, such as regular physical activity, nutritious eating, adequate sleep, and mindfulness or relaxation techniques. A strong foundation of physical health supports mental health recovery.

Pursue Interests and Hobbies: Engaging in activities that bring joy and satisfaction can be a powerful antidote to despair. Encourage individuals to explore new interests or rekindle old passions as a source of hope and fulfillment.

Educating and Advocating

Stay Informed: Keeping up to date with the latest research and developments in schizophrenia treatment can provide hope by highlighting the ongoing progress in understanding and managing the condition.

Advocate for Change: Being part of advocacy efforts for better mental health policies and services not only contributes to societal change but also reinforces a sense of purpose and collective hope.

Embracing Flexibility and Patience

Adapt to Change: Recognize that the journey with schizophrenia involves fluctuations and changes. Being open to adjusting expectations and approaches as needed can help maintain hope in the face of challenges.

Practice Patience: Understanding that progress may be slow and nonlinear helps temper frustrations and setbacks. Patience reinforces the belief that with time and persistence, improvement is achievable.

Highlighting Stories of Hope and Recovery

Share Success Stories: Hearing about others who have successfully navigated the challenges of schizophrenia can be incredibly inspiring. Share these stories within the community to light the way for others.

Conclusion

Fostering hope involves a multifaceted approach that combines practical strategies with emotional support. By celebrating progress, connecting with others, focusing on holistic well-being, staying informed, and embracing flexibility, individuals and families can maintain optimism and forward momentum. This chapter aims to serve as a reminder that, despite the inherent challenges of schizophrenia, there is a path forward filled with potential and promise. The journey is not just about surviving but thriving, propelled by the enduring power of hope.

Conclusion

"The Complete Family Guide to Schizophrenia: Navigating the Journey Together" serves as an invaluable resource for both caregivers and individuals affected by schizophrenia. The book offers comprehensive insights into the complex nature of schizophrenia and provides practical guidance for navigating the challenges that arise along the journey.

One of the strengths of this book is its emphasis on the role of the caregiver in caring for a loved one with schizophrenia. The caregiver's role is pivotal in ensuring the well-being, treatment adherence, and overall quality of life for the individual with schizophrenia. The book highlights the importance of understanding the condition, managing symptoms, promoting treatment and recovery, providing emotional support, and self-care for the caregiver.

By providing a thorough understanding of schizophrenia, the book empowers caregivers to advocate effectively, communicate clearly, and provide appropriate care and support. It addresses the diverse range of symptoms that can arise, such as hallucinations, delusions, disorganized thinking, and impaired behavior and cognition. The book offers strategies and resources for managing these symptoms, ranging from medication management to therapy and coping techniques.

Moreover, the book recognizes the significance of promoting treatment and recovery. It emphasizes the importance of medication adherence, therapy attendance, and engagement in healthy lifestyle choices for the individual with schizophrenia. It encourages caregivers to support their loved ones in finding meaning and purpose through meaningful activities and employment, thus contributing to their overall recovery journey.

"The Complete Family Guide to Schizophrenia" also underscores the crucial role of emotional support for both the caregiver and the individual with schizophrenia. It acknowledges the distressing nature of the illness and provides guidance on how to listen empathetically, validate experiences, and create a safe and supportive environment. The book stresses the importance of open communication and involving the individual in their treatment decisions, fostering a sense of empowerment and autonomy.

In conclusion, "The Complete Family Guide to Schizophrenia: Navigating the Journey Together" is a comprehensive and compassionate guide that equips caregivers with the knowledge and tools needed to care for a loved one with schizophrenia. By addressing key aspects such as understanding the condition, managing symptoms, promoting treatment and recovery, and providing emotional support, this book offers guidance and support for the complex journey of caring for someone with schizophrenia. It serves as a valuable resource for both caregivers and individuals affected by schizophrenia, helping them navigate the challenges they may encounter and fostering hope and resilience along the way.

Resources and Support Networks

Here are some additional resources for families of individuals with schizophrenia:

1. Schizophrenia Research Foundation (India): Provides information, resources, and support for individuals and families affected by schizophrenia in India. Website: https://www.scientificconferences.co.in/srf/index.html

2. Schizophrenia Society of Ontario (Canada): Offers support, education, and advocacy for individuals and families impacted by schizophrenia in Ontario, Canada. Website: https://schizophrenia.on.ca/

3. Schizophrenia and Related Disorders Alliance of America (SARDAA): A non-profit organization that provides support and education for individuals and families affected by schizophrenia and related disorders in the United States. Website: https://sardaa.org/

4. Mental Health America (MHA): Offers a variety of resources, information, and support for individuals and families impacted by mental health conditions, including schizophrenia. Website: https://www.mhanational.org/

5. International Schizophrenia Foundation: A global organization that focuses on increasing awareness, providing education, and supporting research

regarding schizophrenia and related disorders. Website: http://www.mentalhealth.com/

6. SupportGroups.com: An online platform that hosts various support groups, including some specifically for individuals and families affected by schizophrenia. Website: https://www.supportgroups.com/

7. "Schizophrenia and Related Disorders" subreddit: An online community on Reddit where individuals and family members can share experiences, seek support, and find resources related to schizophrenia. The subreddit can be found at: https://www.reddit.com/r/schizophrenia/

Remember, local mental health clinics and hospitals may also have support groups or resources available specifically for families of individuals with schizophrenia. It's always a good idea to reach out to mental health professionals or local healthcare providers for information on additional resources in your specific region.

Here are some schizophrenia family support groups in Australia, Canada, the UK, and the US:

Australia:

1. SANE Australia: Provides information, support, and online forums for individuals and families affected by mental health issues, including schizophrenia. Website: https://www.sane.org/

2. Grow: Offers mutual support groups for individuals and families experiencing mental health challenges,

including schizophrenia. Website:
https://www.grow.org.au/

Canada:

1. Schizophrenia Society of Canada: Provides support, education, and advocacy for individuals and families impacted by schizophrenia. They have local chapters across Canada. Website: https://www.schizophrenia.ca/

2. Canadian Mental Health Association (CMHA): Offers a variety of services and support programs for individuals and families affected by mental health conditions, including schizophrenia. Website: https://cmha.ca/

UK:

1. Rethink Mental Illness: Provides information, advice, and support for individuals and families affected by mental health conditions, including schizophrenia. The organization has local support groups across the UK. Website: https://www.rethink.org/

2. Together for Mental Wellbeing: Offers a wide range of community-based support services, including support for families and carers of individuals with mental health conditions like schizophrenia. Website: https://www.together-uk.org/

US:

1. National Alliance on Mental Illness (NAMI): Provides support, education, and advocacy for individuals and families affected by mental health conditions, including schizophrenia. NAMI has local chapters throughout the United States. Website: https://www.nami.org/

2. Family-to-Family Support Program: A free, evidence-based education program offered by NAMI that provides information, resources, and support for family members of individuals living with schizophrenia and other mental health conditions. Website: https://www.nami.org/Support-Education/Family-to-Family

Please note that support group availability and offerings may vary, so it's recommended to visit the respective websites or contact these organizations directly for more information about local support groups and services in your area.

Glossary of Terms

1. **Schizophrenia:** A severe mental disorder characterized by distortions in thinking, perception, emotions, language, sense of self and behavior.

2. **Psychosis:** A severe mental disorder in which thought and emotions are so impaired that contact is lost with external reality.

3. **Hallucinations:** Sensory experiences that occur in the absence of any actual external stimuli.

4. **Delusions:** Firmly held beliefs that are not based in reality.

5. **Disorganized Speech:** A style of talking often associated with schizophrenia.

6. **Negative Symptoms:** Elements that are 'taken away' from the individual's personality in schizophrenia.

7. **Catatonia:** An abnormal condition variously characterized by stupor, stereotypy, mania, and either rigidity or extreme flexibility of the limbs.

8. **Antipsychotics:** Medications that reduce or relieve symptoms of psychosis.

9. **Cognitive Behavioral Therapy (CBT):** A form of psychotherapy that focuses on the relationships among thoughts, feelings, and behaviors.

10. **Schizoaffective Disorder:** A mental health disorder that is marked by a combination of schizophrenia symptoms and mood disorder symptoms.

11. **Paranoia:** Suspicion and mistrust of people or their actions without evidence or justification.

12. **Anhedonia:** Inability to experience pleasure.

13. **Avolition:** Lack of motivation.

14. **Alogia:** Difficulty in speech.

15. **Flat Affect:** A lack of emotional expression.

16. **Cognitive Deficits:** Impairments in cognitive functions such as memory and attention.

17. **Neuroleptics:** Another term for antipsychotic drugs.

18. **Extrapyramidal Symptoms (EPS):** Side effects such as restlessness, involuntary movements, and muscular tension produced by antipsychotic medication.

19. **Tardive Dyskinesia:** A side effect of long-term use of neuroleptic drugs characterized by involuntary movements.

20. **Psychoeducation:** The process of providing education and information to those seeking or receiving mental health services.

21. **Relapse:** The return of symptoms after a period of improvement.

22. **Remission:** A decrease in or disappearance of signs and symptoms of schizophrenia.

23. **Recovery:** The process of change through which individuals improve their health and wellness, live a self-directed life, and strive to reach their full potential.

24. **Prodromal Symptoms:** Early signs of the onset of an illness.

25. **First Episode Psychosis:** The first time someone experiences psychotic symptoms.

26. **Dual Diagnosis:** The condition of suffering from a mental illness and a comorbid substance abuse problem.

27. **Assertive Community Treatment (ACT):** A team treatment approach designed to provide comprehensive, community-based psychiatric treatment, rehabilitation, and support to persons with serious and persistent mental illness.

28. **Family Therapy:** A type of psychological counseling that can help family members improve communication and resolve conflicts.

29. **Social Skills Training:** Type of behavioral therapy used to improve social skills.

30. **Supported Employment:** Programs that help people with mental health conditions work at regular jobs of their choosing.

31. **Psychiatric Rehabilitation:** A process aimed at recovery from a mental health condition or mental disorder.

32. **Resilience:** The personal strength that helps most people cope with stress and recover from adversity and even trauma.

33. **Stigma:** A mark of disgrace associated with a particular circumstance, quality, or person.

34. **Early Intervention:** A system of services that helps babies and toddlers with developmental delays or disabilities.

35. **Phenothiazines:** A group of antipsychotic drugs used to treat psychotic disorders such as schizophrenia.

36. **Atypical Antipsychotics:** A group of antipsychotic drugs used to treat psychiatric conditions. They are called "atypical" to set them apart from the earlier drugs (the "typical" antipsychotics), which have different side effects.

37. **Typical Antipsychotics:** The first generation of antipsychotic drugs, also known as neuroleptics.

38. **Clozapine:** An atypical antipsychotic medication used to treat severe schizophrenia.

39. **Risperidone:** An atypical antipsychotic drug mainly used to treat schizophrenia.

40. **Olanzapine:** An atypical antipsychotic, used to treat the symptoms of psychotic conditions such as schizophrenia.

41. **Quetiapine:** An antipsychotic medicine that works in the brain to treat schizophrenia.

42. **Aripiprazole:** An atypical antipsychotic used in the treatment of schizophrenia.

43. **Ziprasidone:** An antipsychotic medication used to treat schizophrenia and acute mania or mixed episodes associated with bipolar disorder.

44. **Paliperidone:** An antipsychotic drug used to treat certain mental/mood disorders such as schizophrenia.

45. **Lurasidone:** An atypical antipsychotic used in the treatment of schizophrenia.

46. **Asenapine:** An antipsychotic drug used for the treatment of schizophrenia.

47. **Iloperidone:** An atypical antipsychotic used for the treatment of schizophrenia.

48. **Brexpiprazole:** An atypical antipsychotic used in the treatment of schizophrenia.

49. **Cariprazine:** An antipsychotic medication used in the treatment of schizophrenia.

50. **Lumateperone:** An atypical antipsychotic used for the treatment of schizophrenia.

I hope you find this list helpful! It's worth noting that not all these terms are exclusive to schizophrenia